FLIGHT FOR LIFE

FLIGHT FOR LIFE

An American Company's Dramatic Rescue Of Nigerian Burn Victims

Richard D. Stewart, MD

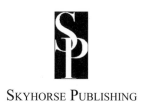

Skyhorse Publishing

Copyright © 2012 by Richard D. Stewart, MD

All Rights Reserved. No part of this book may be reproduced in any manner without the express written consent of the publisher, except in the case of brief excerpts in critical reviews or articles. All inquiries should be addressed to Skyhorse Publishing, 307 West 36th Street, 11th Floor, New York, NY 10018.

Skyhorse Publishing books may be purchased in bulk at special discounts for sales promotion, corporate gifts, fund-raising, or educational purposes. Special editions can also be created to specifications. For details, contact the Special Sales Department, Skyhorse Publishing, 307 West 36th Street, 11th Floor, New York, NY 10018 or info@skyhorsepublishing.com.

Skyhorse® and Skyhorse Publishing® are registered trademarks of Skyhorse Publishing, Inc®, a Delaware corporation.

www.skyhorsepublishing.com

10 9 8 7 6 5 4 3 2 1

Library of Congress Cataloging-in-Publication Data is available on file.

ISBN: 978-1-61608-227-7

Printed in China

For the late patriarch whose philosophy of life and business ethics
set the stage for this dramatic rescue mission—
Samuel C. "Sam" Johnson, chairman emeritus of Johnson Wax,
who died of cancer in May 2004 at age seventy-four.

CONTENTS

Preface xi

Prologue — Disaster Strikes:
Lagos, Nigeria—Monday, June 12, 1982 xiii

Chapter 1 — The Calm before the Storm: Racine,
Wisconsin—Tuesday, 5:47 AM 1

Chapter 2 — Setting Things in Motion:
Racine—Tuesday, 9:15 AM 9

Chapter 3 — Can We Get the Help We Need?
Racine—Tuesday, 10:15 AM 23

Chapter 4 — We're on the Way:
O'Hare International Airport,
Chicago—Tuesday, 6:00 PM 37

Chapter 5 — We Have a Bit of a Problem, Gentlemen:
London—Wednesday, 9:05 AM 43

Chapter 6 — Arriving at the Scene:
Lagos—Thursday, 9:00 AM 53

Chapter 7 — No African Hospitals Can Help:
Lagos—Thursday, Noon 61

Chapter 8 — Can We Get Help from Europe?
Lagos—Thursday Afternoon 73

Contents

Chapter 9	Plan B: Lagos—Thursday Evening	81
Chapter 10	Looking for Miracles: London—Friday, 3:00 AM	87
Chapter 11	Martinair to the Rescue: Lagos—Saturday, 2:00 AM	93
Chapter 12	More Delays: Lagos—Saturday, Noon	109
Chapter 13	Over the Atlantic: Saturday Afternoon and Evening	117
Chapter 14	Touchdown in Detroit, Michigan: Saturday, 9:15 PM	129
Chapter 15	Ann Arbor, Michigan: Sunday Morning	137
Chapter 16	Hoping for Miracles: Ann Arbor—Sunday Afternoon	147
Chapter 17	Ann Arbor: One Week Later	155
Chapter 18	A Visitor from Nigeria: Ann Arbor—July and August	161
Chapter 19	The Final Hurdle: Ann Arbor—Nine Months Later	171

Afterword 177

Acknowledgments 183

Bibliography and Notes 185

About the Author 187

In the twilight of a doctor's life, it's a joy to remember
the thrilling adventures of saving those
who desperately needed medical care.
R. D. S.

PREFACE

Flight for Life is the story of one of the most hair-raising rescue missions in African history. It was a *first*—the first time up until 1982 that an American company showed their extreme dedication to their employees by actively trying to save the lives of twenty-two severely burned Nigerian employees at an overseas subsidiary company because in all of Africa there were no burn care facilities.

The events that prompted SC Johnson's executives to send a rescue mission to Nigeria in an attempt to actively help save the lives of its overseas employees is nonetheless remarkable and should stand as an example of what all powerful corporations the world over should be willing to do in times of internal crisis. Twenty-eight years have passed since this life-changing event, yet there have never been any self-congratulatory declarations made by the eight key participants who helped in the rescue mission. Five of these executives are in the twilight of their lives; three have died. As a primary witness and a physician, who is also in the twilight of his life, I feel compelled to tell this unique, once-in-a-century humanitarian story—precisely how it began; how lives were saved; what the economic costs were; what the survivors' lives are like today; and, from my vantage point the most intriguing aspect of the tale, the personal lives and achievements of the key participants, pre- and post-1982, that motivated them to act as they did.

As the medical officer for SC Johnson during the time of this story, I felt compelled to take notes and photographs. I also recorded the daily action into a portable Dictaphone. I have included actual dialogue only where I was able to confirm it with the people involved. Using my notes and recordings, this is how I recall the events of this episode in our history.

Richard D. Stewart, MD
June 2011

PROLOGUE

Disaster Strikes: Lagos, Nigeria— Monday, June 12, 1982

7:00 AM. It is the season of rain and sweltering summer heat. Occasional lightning flashes strike and illuminate the low-lying dark clouds that hover over the streets of Lagos. The seventy-eight rain-gear-clad employees of Johnson–Nigeria, including three executives, cling to umbrellas and hurry to take shelter inside the walls of their modern factory situated within an industrial park complex.

9:00 AM. Rising water begins to clog the street drains in the area and becomes over a foot deep. Within the Johnson plant, drains are starting to overflow.

10:45 AM. The rains become much heavier. The plant's gashouse operator reports a dangerously high water level in the building. He asks Oli One, the thirty-seven-year-old operations manager, to come and evaluate the situation.

10:50 AM. When Oli One observes the rising water, he gives the order to stop filling the commercial product

Flight for Life

containers but to continue the water bath testing for any leaks in the units that had already been filled. All but five gashouse employees are dispatched to work in other areas until the rising waters recede.

11:40 AM. Inside the plant, the maintenance supervisor and the products superintendent nervously peer out at the driving rain, concerned that the rising floodwaters may collapse the eight-foot-high cement boundary wall spanning the north side of the facility. The wall, which serves as a barrier to the adjacent undeveloped property, protects the Johnson gas and solvent pipelines located a few feet aboveground just inside the perimeter. Joined by four other workers, the two men don their rain gear and wade through the now two-foot-deep water to inspect the wall; but what they most fear happens—water spurts through large widening cracks in the wall. The maintenance supervisor splashes through mid-calf-deep water up to the wall and notes that the floodwater on the other side has risen to a height of five feet. Collapse of the wall appears imminent.

11:43 AM. The maintenance supervisor splashes through the rising water to notify Oli One of the crisis.

11:44 AM. Oli One rushes up to the second floor of the main building and bursts into the office of Allison Ehiemere, the forty-one-year-old general manager, to inform him of the impending disaster. Ehiemere and several other executives hurry outside to assess the damage and potential danger.

11:45 AM. Wading in rapidly rising water, Ehiemere and the executives see a section of the boundary wall suddenly collapse and release a deluge of floodwater into the Johnson compound. They watch in horror as the butane-and-solvent pipelines adjacent to the wall bend, then snap, followed by the hiss of escaping gas. Bursting bubbles give birth to a dense and rapidly expanding vapor cloud of butane gas and flammable solvents that fills the compound. Stunned employees glance at one another, fearful that a lightning strike could ignite the cloud into a flaming coffin. Ehiemere notes that the electrical cables adjacent to the broken pipelines are now submerged in two feet of water, and he fears that the ignition of the vapor cloud could cause a catastrophic explosion. Should the forty-ton butane tank feeding the broken pipeline ignite and explode, the entire industrial park in which Johnson–Nigeria resides could be destroyed.

11:46 AM. Technicians rush to disconnect the electrical power and close all the pipeline valves.

11:47 AM. A series of lightning flashes illuminate the grounds as a worker closes the electrical switches, but unfortunately, he is too late. The dense vapor cloud that fills the area bursts into a massive fireball. "God help me!" Ehiemere screams as he dives beneath the surface of the knee-deep rising pool of water in which he is standing. Twenty-nine employees who are wading in the water scream in pain as they are instantly engulfed in the fireball. Their clothes ignite, and the intensity of the heat burns and blisters their exposed skin. They are surrounded by small pools of flaming solvent floating on the surface of the water. The current sweeps these flaming pools toward the Johnson buildings.

11:48 AM. The entire fiberglass roof of the gashouse melts. The driving rain pours through the gaping hole and quickly extinguishes the steam hissing from the pools of the melted fiberglass. Having nothing more to feed on, the fireball vanishes in a cloud of dark smoke.

11:49 AM. Ehiemere, whose face, hands, and arms are seriously burned, screams out for someone to help the victims travel to one of the four hospitals in the area. He then orders someone to rush him, along with several employees, to the small Ajanaku Hospital, with which the company has a contractual arrangement for the health care of its employees.

Typical of all Nigerian businesses in the early '80s, the only telephone available to the employees to call for help is located some miles away in the private home of Ehiemere.

11:50 AM. Jim Keane, the corporate vice president of international marketing who is visiting from the United States, sees the fireball catastrophe from the second-story window of the adjacent main office. As the burn victims are being helped into cars to be taken to area hospitals, he asks Mr. Fowode, one of the surviving Nigerian executives, to drive him to the hospitals so he could learn how badly the victims were burned.

12:30 PM. By the time the Municipal Fire Brigade arrives around forty-five minutes after the fire began, the surviving employees have extinguished all the flames.

1:00 PM. Keane and Fowode, now the acting general manager, arrive at the first hospital, where the temperature is well over ninety degrees Fahrenheit; the relative humidity is 100 percent. There is no air-conditioning, and no fans are in operation. The electricity is off, a common daily occurrence in Lagos. There is no backup generator. A doctor leads the two men to one of the bedsides in the crowded room. They see a young woman—a secretary and mother of four children—who is heavily sedated and appears to be pain-free. A nurse is busily wrapping gauze bandages around the woman's body to cover the hideous full-thickness-degree burns that cover over 36 percent of her body.

The doctor then leads Keane and Fowode to the bedsides of the other burn victims. Most have sustained more extensive burns than the young woman. All have been heavily sedated, but their burned flesh has not been thoroughly washed or cleaned.

The victims are all in a crowded ward filled with patients, some of whom are suffering from various life-threatening infectious diseases. Keane, who, before joining SC Johnson eight years earlier, had extensive marketing and medical experience with other companies, asks why they aren't being cared for in a sterile intensive care facility as full-thickness skin burns can be lethal once infection sets in. He is told the hospital has no such unit, nor does it have private rooms.

At the second hospital, Keane and Fowode are told that the burns of the patients are so severe that all will probably die. They receive the same bleak prognosis at the third hospital. When Keane asks why, the doctors lament that the hospitals lack the facilities, *intravenous* fluids, and antibiotics to properly care for patients with far less serious burns—burns that would not be lethal in Nigeria if a burn center and the essential medical supplies were available. The best the Nigerian doctors can do with the medicines and equipment they have is to keep badly burned patients *comfortable until death*. It is known that no one survives a large, skin-deep burn in Nigeria.

Keane is then informed that all the larger U.S. and European companies who have businesses located in Nigeria are only obligated to pay the family of any worker who is accidentally killed on the job $5,000, and nothing more.

Keane insists that he must immediately notify those at SC Johnson who might be able to rectify this nightmarish situation. He asks Mr. Fowode to find a driver to take him to a major European-owned plant in the area from which he sends a wire telex message to the Johnson corporate headquarters in Racine, Wisconsin, requesting the services of a U.S. physician and medical supplies. Next he calls London to notify the two top Johnson executives responsible for Nigeria—Barney Miller, the vice president and regional director for Africa and the Near East, and Victor Thomas, the area director for most of the African countries and those in the Near East.

4:00 PM. While Keane does what he can to rectify the hideous situation and escape from this nightmare, Johnson–Nigeria's acting general manager calmly begins to notify the immediate families of the burn victims that the lives of their loved ones are in jeopardy and that they may soon depart the earth.

CHAPTER 1

The Calm before the Storm: Racine, Wisconsin—Tuesday, 5:47 AM

I slipped into my jogging outfit, did my warm-up exercises, and began the two-and-a-half-mile jog along the shores of Lake Michigan. Overhead a solitary seagull was soaring in large circles against the cloudless blue of the morning sky. A faint breeze ruffled the tips of the waves, causing sparkles of sunlight to be reflected as the waves rolled toward the shore. The tranquil beauty surrounding me sent my spirits soaring.

As I jogged, with the stirring melodies of *The Sound of Music* resonating through my Walkman, I daydreamed about the future—writing a new chapter on high-altitude sickness for Harper & Row's *Practice of Medicine* (for which I was one of the editors); creating a new sequence of teaching slides on toxicology to better engage my medical students, interns, and residents; and, to top the list, planning a wilderness canoe and camping trip in northern Wisconsin with my wife, Mary—the love of my life—and our thirteen-year-old daughter, Beth, the only one of our three children still living at home.

As a fifty-five-year-old physician, all was right in my world. Seven days earlier, I had joyously celebrated my thirtieth wedding anniversary by dancing until midnight with the lady who for me had the most spontaneous smile and enthralling deep blue eyes of any creature on the planet. In the field of medicine, my true academic love, I was entering my sixteenth year as a professor of internal medicine and medical toxicology at the Medical College of Wisconsin, Milwaukee; and I was in my fifth year as the corporate medical director of SC Johnson, a large American corporation that got its start making Johnson Wax and graduating into other household chemical products. In that role, I had two main responsibilities—overseeing product toxicology and establishing a model emergency and preventive medicine facility for its three thousand U.S. employees. I had absolutely no responsibility for and little knowledge about the fifty-four foreign Johnson subsidiaries, including the one in Nigeria. In fact, all I knew about Nigeria in 1982 was that it was an oil-rich African country plagued by political unrest and economic distress, as reported in *Time* magazine and *The Wall Street Journal*.

That morning I had no inkling that the telephone call I was about to receive would interrupt the serenity in which I was basking and propel me into the most hair-raising medical adventure of my career. After breakfast—on what was to prove to be an unforgettable day—I drove four miles

The Calm before the Storm: Racine, Wisconsin—Tuesday, 5:47 AM

to the Johnson Medical Center, which was situated in building 43E in the heart of the Johnson production and shipping complex located on a large plot of land on the western fringe of Racine. I parked and hurried up the concrete steps leading to the building's inviting entrance with its huge glass doors. Inside, the center was bustling with activity. All the nurses were smiling, a good sign that everything was running on schedule. The ER suite was empty—another good sign. As I passed the reception area on the way to my office, I saw several employees busily updating their medical histories prior to their annual examination.

SC Johnson, at the time, was one of the world's leading manufacturers of chemical specialty products for home, auto, and personal use as well as for commercial maintenance and industrial markets. The majority of the company's stock was privately owned by the family, and its profits were rumored to be astronomical during bull markets.

I had been working for the company for ten years. In 1972, Sam Johnson, the CEO and holder of the majority of the stock of the private multinational company, invited me to use the consulting time I was allowed by the Medical College of Wisconsin to oversee their product toxicology operation. At the time, all I knew about the Racine facility was that it was privately owned and that the building was a Frank Lloyd Wright design.

During our get-to-know-each-other session, Sam Johnson and I were seated in comfortable chairs in his ultramodern office. For me this was a unique experience. Sam Johnson was the first billionaire with whom I had ever conversed. He was a muscular balding fifty-four-year-old gentleman with a warm smile and sparkling blue eyes. He was dressed in a dark gray business suit and wore comfortable-looking black loafers. During our conversation, I learned that both of us had enlisted in the U.S. Air Force and had qualified for pilot training. Apparently, we both wanted the thrill of soaring high above the earth in the vast freedom of the sky.

Luckily, I had qualified for pilot training at seventeen at Keesler Field near Biloxi, Mississippi, three months before World War II ended. Born on March 2, 1928, Sam had earned a bachelor's degree in economics from Cornell University and an MBA from Harvard Business School before enlisting in the U.S. Air Force and qualifying for pilot training. At seventeen, Sam had learned to fly and did so for the rest of his life. He served as a first lieutenant and intelligence officer but did not see combat. Discharged in 1954, he joined the family company then headed by his father, H. F. Johnson Jr.

In 1967, Sam became chairman of the SC Johnson & Son Inc. and turned the $171-million wax company into a thriving, multibillion-dollar family-owned empire of four global companies employing close to 13,000 people, excluding the temporary workers. This was accomplished in large measure by his business strategy and creation of a new products development group that introduced successful brands like Glade™, Raid™, and Pledge™ into the marketplace. His business strategy was simple: new products, new geographics, and every few years, an acquisition.

The history of the SC Johnson company is progressive and impressive. In 1886, a salesman named Samuel C. Johnson—Sam's great-grandfather—began manufacturing parquet floors in the rear of his hardware store in Racine. The business flourished, and after two years, he introduced

The Calm before the Storm: Racine, Wisconsin—Tuesday, 5:47 AM

a new product into the market—paste wax. The demand for the wax soared, leading Johnson to establish a new company, SC Johnson & Son (also known as Johnson Wax). The company expanded, and with over 13,000 employees worldwide by 1982, it established itself as one of the world's leading manufacturers of chemical specialty products for homes, autos, personal care, insect control, and industrial maintenance.

Sam personally conducted my first tour of the Johnson facilities. The automation of the production lines and the contented attitude of the employees were impressive. I learned later from the head of personnel that SC Johnson had similar highly automated facilities in many countries around the world, including Nigeria, Japan, and China. I also learned that all employees not only received above-standard union wages but were also participants in the annual Christmas profit-sharing extravaganza.

The only unexpected surprise during that first tour occurred when I glanced inside the nursing station that served as the sole medical facility. The primary duty of the two nurses was to fit safety glasses and work shoes for all employees. All accidental injuries and illnesses were referred to the workers' personal physicians, few of whom had any training in product toxicology or occupational medicine. As we walked away from the nursing station, I boldly told Sam that the nursing station was a small blemish on such a technologically advanced firm. As I saw it, in the category of employee health, SC Johnson was fifteen years behind the national norm.

I could tell that my remark had wounded Sam and cast a pall over what had been a remarkably pleasant morning. By the end of our tour, Sam offered me a consulting salary three times greater than the Medical College of Wisconsin would allow. I told him that while I would relish the toxicology challenge, I could only accept one-third of the offered consulting fee.

Sam told me he would give me the balance of his offer in unrestricted grants for research I wished to do while at the medical college. I had previously invented a number of medical devices and introduced them into medicine, including the Silastic intravenous catheter, an artificial capillary lung, and the hollow fiber artificial kidney. At the time of our meeting, I was heading a research team studying the human absorption, metabolism, excretion, and physiologic/pharmacologic responses to thirty-two toxic agents commonly encountered in the workplace.

I was delighted with Sam's consultation offer, and we sealed the deal with a handshake. Several days later, the "simple" task of designing, building, and staffing a model medical facility to care for all three thousand U.S. employees was added to my consulting duties. I wrestled with this startling pronouncement for a few minutes and concluded that no company with only three thousand U.S. employees could afford the "model medical facility" I had been asked to establish. However, I submitted a grand plan fashioned after what I had observed at the Dow Chemical Company in Midland, Michigan, and at the Mayo Clinic in Rochester, Minnesota. The main emphasis was on preventive medicine measures—periodic comprehensive physical examinations focused on the early detection of potentially serious diseases such as diabetes, obesity, coronary heart disease, and cancer.

The Calm before the Storm: Racine, Wisconsin—Tuesday, 5:47 AM

Ideally, the medical facility would feature a gymnasium and indoor pool. Included was a system for computerizing each employee's medical records along with periodic measurements of their exposures to toxic chemical agents in the workplace.

That evening, while my wife and I enjoyed dinner, I expounded that my plan would most certainly be rejected due to the cost. The next day, though, to my complete astonishment, Sam not only agreed to build the facility but also asked that I recruit the necessary doctors, nurses, and personnel to staff it. Only then did I fully realize SC Johnson's inclusive business philosophy—a philosophy that trumped many of the other larger U.S. corporate firms. At SC Johnson, all employees, I determined, were respected profit-sharing partners.

For my first six years at the company, I oversaw product toxicology while serving as the part-time corporate medical advisor. Then, in 1978, I joined SC Johnson as its first full-time corporate medical director, responsible for U.S. operations. While performing these duties, I was still granted 20 percent of my time to continue my research and teaching at the Medical College of Wisconsin—a privilege I have always cherished.

CHAPTER 2

Setting Things in Motion: Racine—Tuesday, 9:15 AM

Twenty-seven hours after the butane gas explosion and fireball occurred in Nigeria, as I was sorting through the mail and the telephone requests that had piled up during my brief absence from the office, I received a call from Roger Mulhollen, vice president of human relations at SC Johnson who told me that late yesterday they received a telex from Jim Keane, vice president of marketing international consumer products, who was visiting our company in Nigeria.

When I said I knew Jim, Mulhollen told me that Jim was requesting the assistance of an American physician and the essential medical supplies to treat as many as thirty-three Nigerian employees who had been seriously burned in a butane gas explosion at our plant. They had no idea how many of the burns were serious. Mulhollen paused a moment and told me that Bob Peterson had asked him to relay it to me. L. Robert "Bob" Peterson was the vice president of international consumer products and the top senior executive at SC Johnson directly responsible for consumer products in the foreign countries in which the company was involved.

It struck me that sending a message like this one was a strange move on the part of Jim Keane. I knew the man; he was a clever entrepreneur—a businessman with a broad smile who never acted erratically. If faced with a major medical problem in Nigeria, he would certainly have asked the general manager of Johnson–Nigeria to consult with the doctors in that country.

"That's it," I asked Mulhollen, wondering why I was being informed. Mulhollen told me that Jim Keane wanted the assistance of an American physician and all the essential medical supplies to care for thirty or so seriously burned employees. That was all he knew.

The fact of the matter was I had no medical responsibility for the employees at the Nigerian plant. I concluded that Nigerian physicians would certainly know what best to do in the event of an industrial accident. Furthermore, Nigeria had a fine university medical school with a world-renowned hospital located in Lagos. I completely believed they'd be fully capable of handling patient care for burned people.

"Where is the Johnson plant in Nigeria located?" I queried, hoping it was near the capital. When Mulhollen said it was in Lagos, I was completely puzzled. *Why would Jim Keane, a visiting corporate executive from Racine, make such a request, especially when there was a first-class hospital in the same city?* I wondered. I asked to speak directly with Keane to obtain more details about the situation unfolding across the globe but was told it was not possible. They had been trying but were unable to reach Keane by telephone. For one of the wealthiest nations in Africa, Nigeria had about the poorest telephone communication system in the world at the time. It was easy to make a call in the country but at times impossible to reach someone in it.

I decided to call Bob Peterson and see if he had instructions for me. My curiosity was piqued, and I assumed that Peterson was going to ask me to be the one to journey to Nigeria—a country I had no real desire to visit—to assess the situation. Without delay, I dialed Peterson's office and asked to speak with him.

Peterson was a stout well-built man a few years older than I who had a smile and a sales pitch that few could resist. He had served in the U.S. Army from 1943 through 1945, experiencing some real adventures with the Thirteenth Armored Division in Europe, including the Battle of the Bulge. After discharge as a staff sergeant, he had enrolled at the University of Wisconsin, interested in business. In 1947, he worked for SC Johnson as a salesman in Madison, Wisconsin, after which he had risen swiftly through the ranks to become the top sales executive for Johnson International. Johnson–Nigeria was one of the companies in his bailiwick.

Suddenly Peterson's deep voice boomed over the phone, and he told me he was glad I was in the office today because we had a big problem. I asked if he was talking about Keane's request for a doctor and supplies. He said he was, but that was just the tip of the iceberg. I told him to go ahead, I was all ears.

Peterson explained that a little after ten o'clock the previous morning, he received a call from Barney Miller in London. He was the vice president and regional director for Africa and the Near East. Peterson reminded me that while

I may remember Miller as the company's in-house guitar player and comedian, he was unsurpassed as the manager of the overseas operations. Barney gave Peterson the bad news that flooding had collapsed a retaining wall on the plant perimeter and severed a gas pipeline. All the valves to the pipeline were immediately turned off, but somehow an electrical spark or a lightning strike ignited the escaping cloud of butane gas, causing a massive explosion. Thirty-five or so employees were burned—twenty-two badly—including the general manager, the product manager, and the financial manager.

Peterson told me that he learned more around 2:00 PM our time—8:00 PM in Nigeria—when Jim Keane called him directly about the catastrophe. Miller told him that everyone had moved so fast it was unbelievable. The uninjured employees quickly extinguished the fires throughout the plant and rushed the burn victims to four different hospitals. Keane and the new acting general manager had visited over half of the burn victims and were on the way to check on the rest. Miller said it was pretty awful. The doctors told him that Nigerian hospitals lacked the antibiotics and IV fluids necessary to treat burn patients, and that most of the employees would die. That is why Jim made his request for help.

Peterson said he didn't hear any more until eight thirty this morning when Vic Thomas, the area director responsible for Nigeria who reports directly to Miller, sent him a telex from London. Petersen read me the telex in which Thomas said he was leaving for Lagos to take stock of the situation. After he and Keane talked, they agreed that Nigeria lacked proper medical supplies for serious burn cases and they would need help from medical personnel in Racine, who would be more familiar with the types of burns caused by an LPG explosion. They wanted us to send essential medical supplies and, hopefully, a visit to Nigeria by one of the company doctors.

I had met Vic Thomas and his wife once before at one of Johnson's international conferences. I remembered him as a towering Nigerian who spoke impeccable English, and his wife was from England. What I wish I had known about the man was that Vic's father, Dr. Horatio Oritsejolomi Thomas, had been one of the most revered physicians and surgeons in all of Nigeria. *Oritisejolomi* in the Itsekiri language means "God has put me on earth to do good works."

When Peterson asked me what I thought, I hardly knew where to start. First of all, I did not know the quality of the medical care that the Nigerian employees were now receiving or what was available for burn patients in that country. Peterson responded with a remark that stunned me. He told me to believe him, that the medical care in Nigeria was rotten. This remark stunned me—*rotten medical care in Nigeria?* It couldn't be true.

I asked about the university hospital in Lagos, staffed by well-trained doctors who should know how best to treat burn patients. Peterson told me he had seen that hospital and that it was situated right in the middle of a marsh teeming with mosquitoes carrying malaria. He told me it was a hellhole— that the government didn't give them enough money for medicine or staff and that people only went there to die.

I sensed that Peterson had fired a "you are on your way to Nigeria" missile and that it was headed straight for me. Were I to duck, I had better come up with the name of a burn specialist or two—someone from a burn center in

England, France, or Germany. When I asked if he was suggesting that I go to Lagos and check things out, he said he was not suggesting, he was asking. He told me that as the company's top doctor, he wanted me to assess the situation and advise them what best to do. I told him I was not a specialist in the treatment of burns, and he quickly countered that I must have taken care of burns before.

It was true that I had treated burns before, but I hesitated momentarily, stalling until I could come up with a better solution to this situation. I remembered the seriously burned workers at the Dow Chemical Company in Midland, Michigan, whom I had seen and helped care for in 1958 and again in 1964. The dying gasps of two of such patients with 100 percent total body burns was a recurrent nightmarish memory for me.

Assuming I was taking on the challenge, Peterson told me that once I got to Lagos and assessed the situation, I could then advise SC Johnson about what additional measures, if any, they should take. Peterson's missile was nearing its target. I told him that if there were badly burned employees in need of medical supplies, that time was of the essence. The first twenty-four hours were the most critical in burn care, and if the treatment has been poor, the outcome will be disastrous—and we were already twenty-four hours behind in knowing what had been done.

Peterson asked me directly if I would go. I paused a moment, unable to think of another option. It would require time we didn't have to search for a burn specialist who would drop everything and rush to Nigeria. When he pushed me for a yes or no, I finally agreed. With the decision made I told him the sooner I got to Lagos the better. I couldn't believe

Setting Things in Motion: Racine—Tuesday, 9:15 AM

I was committing myself to this task, but, after all, I was the senior Johnson physician in the United States.

Peterson asked me if I had a valid passport and I told him I did. I sensed I was pushing my medical canoe into some white-water rapids where I might not only lose the canoe but have to swim for my life. Africa was a cesspool of infectious diseases—yellow fever, cholera, schistosomiasis, and guinea worms that would squirm in your intestines. Malaria was rampant and a major killer. If I made a quick trip to Nigeria today, I wouldn't have the time to begin the mandatory two-week malaria preventative protection with chloroquine.

Peterson told me I'd need a visa and that could be a bit tricky because it could take up to three weeks to obtain unless there was a direct invitation from the Nigerian government. I reminded him that we would already have lost at least three critical days if counting the time it will take to fly there. I reminded him that if some of the badly burned employees haven't received the proper treatment—IV fluids, antibiotics, wound cleansing in a clean environment—my visiting them after three days have elapsed makes this a worthless trip; all the seriously burned will need is a priest for last rites and burial.

A lot of the Nigerians are Muslims and I had never before dealt with a seriously ill patient who was Muslim. It concerned me since I wasn't sure what ceremony to follow if one of these patients should die. The white-water rapids were filled not only with rocks that could rip the bottom out of my canoe but with alligators as well.

Still on the phone, Peterson told me he thought we may be able to work out obtaining a vias quickly with a letter of intent addressed to the Nigerian government, signed by a company officer, and presented to the Nigerians by none other than Sam Johnson's cousin, John Louis Jr., our nation's ambassador to Great Britain. In anticipation of the visa problem, Peterson told me he had called Louis earlier that morning and was assured that I would be able to enter Lagos from London. And Barney Miller would then meet me at the London airport and take me to the U.S. Embassy to meet with Ambassador Louis, who would arrange the immediate entry into Nigeria.

Peterson told me we were ahead of the game in one area. He had already taken the liberty to check out flight schedules and there were some late-afternoon flights to Lagos that day. He told me to go home and get packed for a week's stay in tropical Africa. He said he would get the tickets and the money I would need and that his secretary would call me at home with all the arrangements. Unless things changed dramatically, he asked that I plan on meeting him in his office after lunch at two o'clock to speak with him and Ray Farley and he told me to invite Bill Eastham.

Raymond F. Farley was the president and chief operating officer of SC Johnson at the time. In his fifties, he boasted a tall, athletic build, evidence that he still exercised regularly. I understood that in his younger days, he had been a varsity letter winner at Northwestern University.

William Eastham was the man to whom I now reported. He was Johnson's former president and chief operating officer, and in his departing year at the company, he was serving as the vice chairman. Bill had always been highly supportive of my human toxicology studies. During World War II, he had served on General George Patton's staff, and he hadn't lost any of his dynamic approach in coping with a problem.

Setting Things in Motion: Racine—Tuesday, 9:15 AM

I dialed Eastham's number. His secretary answered and offered to take a message. Bill was attending a board of directors meeting. I told her I was facing a company medical emergency and that it was imperative that I speak with him immediately. She found him and soon he was speaking gruffly into the receiver asking me what I wanted. Eastham sounded like a general addressing one of his lieutenants as he spoke on the phone. I informed him of Keane's request for a U.S. physician and medical supplies to attend to the patients in Nigeria.

Eastham said he knew that Jim wouldn't ask for something like that unless there was a good reason to. He knew Jim Keane was no dummy when it came to the practice of medicine. He spent several years as the group product manager with the Bristol-Myers company and as the vice president of advertising and product management with the Warner-Lambert Company.

I recalled that Keane did possess an ardent interest in medicine. On several occasions, he had queried me as to my opinion about several over-the-counter medications that Johnson might consider marketing. He viewed the OTC arena as a promising one for Johnson to enter. The man knew medicine, no doubt about it.

I explained that Bob Peterson wanted me to go to Lagos and assess the situation as soon as possible. Without hesitation, Eastham said he agreed completely. He told me to go and not to waste any time getting there.

"Right now I don't know what medical supplies are needed—which ones or in what quantity," I said.

Communication with anyone in Africa could be a big problem, Eastham explained. He told me that Jim knew this, and when facing an emergency in Nigeria, he would go to the U.S. Embassy for help because they possessed the best communication system in Africa. He paused, and in a commanding voice told me to remember that the U.S. Embassy was there if I needed help. He told me to let him know if I needed any help for anything, such as a ride to O'Hare International Airport. He said he would put the company helicopter on standby so if I had to make a mad dash to O'Hare, it would be available.

I was impressed with the speed with which the Johnson hierarchy was going all out to respond to the Nigerian call for help before they knew how much help would be needed or what it might cost. I took several deep breaths to relax. This promised to be another of my bucking-bronco adventures in medicine. I prayed I could stay in the saddle and accomplish the mission. There was a lot to do and precious little time in which to do it.

The next call I made was to my wife, Mary. Our home phone rang about a dozen times before I heard a "hello" followed by several quick breaths. It was my daughter, Beth, and I could picture her hobbling on crutches due to her recent knee surgery in an effort to reach the telephone.

"Beth, please let me speak with your mom."

"Mom's not here. She's grocery shopping."

I felt urgent in my request. "When she returns, please tell her that I'm flying to Nigeria later today and that I could use her help packing."

"You're kidding me, right?"

"No, I'm really going. Just tell her, Beth. I'll be coming home soon."

I thought about what little I did know of Nigeria. Equal in size to the combined areas of California, Utah, and Nevada,

Setting Things in Motion: Racine—Tuesday, 9:15 AM

Nigeria's population of 115 million—the largest in Africa as of the early 1980s—was distributed among more than 250 tribal groups, each with a different dialect. I remembered reading that Nigeria was granted full independence from Great Britain in 1960, inheriting a parliamentary representative government from the British. English remained the official national language, so at least once I was in the country, communication with the medical staff and patients shouldn't pose a problem. But beyond that, my knowledge of the African nation was very slim, though I realized this would not be the biggest hurdle I'd have to overcome once in the country.

The biggest problem, I determined, would be the festering internal unrest within the country. The discovery of huge oil reserves in 1956 catapulted the country into the role of the richest nation in Africa. A small number of the wealthy elite and a clique of military officers with unbridled access to Nigeria's multibillion-dollar oil-exporting business had amassed fortunes. However, the standard of living for the general public hadn't improved appreciably, and poverty remained widespread. The military came to power in a coup d'état in 1966 and suspended the constitution. Finally, in 1979, civilian rule was restored, and a new constitution established a government closely resembling that of the United States, with a president and vice president elected every four years, a legislature similar to ours, and an independent judiciary.

Dee Becker, my secretary, rushed into my office and handed me two messages. One informed me that Vic Thomas was preparing to depart for Lagos and was requesting I call him at his home in London. The other was from Paul Bodeau, a Johnson engineer and industrial hygienist who was apparently familiar with the Nigerian plant.

I asked Dee to place the first call to Vic. I informed him that before I could respond to the request for medical supplies, I needed to know the number of burn patients, the severity of each one's burns, and the medical supplies currently available in the local hospitals. Vic thanked me for coming and informed me that he would meet me upon my arrival at the Lagos airport, then drive me to the Graz Hotel, Anthony Village, Lagos, where he had taken the liberty to make room reservations for the two of us. Once I had visited the patients, he would do his best to procure what I judged to be the essential medical supplies.

During our brief conversation, it occurred to me that it would be an excellent move on my part if I could be accompanied by a bona fide expert in the treatment of severe burns. The major obstacle was finding one on such short notice. The only burn specialist I knew personally was Dr. Irving Feller, the medical director of the Burn Program and the chief of the Division of Burn Surgery at the University of Michigan. I decided it was worth the gamble to give him a quick call.

I knew Irv had written several books on the treatment of burns. To stay updated on the latest developments in burn therapy, I perused several of them at the University of Michigan Medical School library a few years back. If and when I got into a debate with the Nigerian doctors, having one of Dr. Feller's books tucked under my arm would be fine, but having Dr. Feller along would be a godsend.

I called the University of Michigan Medical Center hotline and was transferred to the Burn Center. Irv's wife, Cynthia, who was in charge of patient scheduling, answered.

"Burn Center Scheduling, Cynthia Feller speaking. How may I help you?"

Setting Things in Motion: Racine—Tuesday, 9:15 AM

"This is Dr. Richard Stewart. I'm the corporate medical director for SC Johnson in Racine, Wisconsin. We have an urgent need for a consultation. May I please speak with Dr. Feller?" I paused and emphasized, "This is an emergency."

"Dr. Feller is in surgery right now. Would you kindly tell me about the emergency so I can relay your request to Dr. Feller?"

"Please tell him that Dick Stewart, an old colleague of his, called and that I wish for him to serve as a consultant for thirty or so recently burned patients in Nigeria." I quickly sketched out the details of what I knew about the Nigerian affair, managing to slip into our conversation a comment or two about my intermittent but long-term relationship with Irv. She was most gracious and told me that she would personally hand-deliver my message to Dr. Feller in the operating room. In closing she did warn me that during the summer break he was booked solid performing plastic surgery necessary to restore a more normal appearance for children with disfiguring burn scars, so it was highly unlikely he would be able to consult at this time, especially overseas. I hung up and feared that just as I had anticipated, Irv was far too committed to journey to Nigeria on such short notice.

I quickly called Paul Bodeau, the corporate safety manager. He gave me his theoretical appraisal of the explosion, telling me that the open-air fireball probably didn't possess the potential to do much physical damage to the plant. From the information he had been able to gather, only one person whose shirt had caught fire was seriously burned. This gave me pause, and after I hung up, I debated the wisdom of rushing a burn expert away from his seriously ill patients to Nigeria only to see *one* serious burn patient.

It was a short debate, and I decided in favor of Jim Keane, the man on the spot who had observed multiple burn victims in the four hospitals. If Irv could be persuaded to join me, I would take him along.

Shortly after 10:30 AM, I closed my office, knowing I would be facing real misery upon my return. There was an ongoing product toxicology research project that needed my daily surveillance while a critical overdue manuscript also needed editing. Both were going to be severely neglected.

CHAPTER 3

Can We Get the Help We Need?
Racine—Tuesday, 10:15 AM

A series of potential problems began to surface as I drove the fifteen-minute commute to our home on Wind Point Road. I knew nothing about the insect control or the sanitation where I would be staying in Nigeria—disturbing thoughts for me. Until I learned precisely what I was facing, I had better go prepared for the worst-possible scenario, I decided. I would treat the upcoming stay in Africa as I had my multiple one-month stays as a medical missionary in the lowlands of Bolivia and the northern provinces of Argentina studying Chagas' disease, the parasitic heart and neurological disease. The insecticides and medicines I had used kept me healthy in a few of the deadliest parasite- and mosquito-infested regions of the world, so the same protective measures would almost undoubtedly keep me safe in Africa—I would only drink boiled or chlorinated water, and all my food would also have to first be washed in the same water.

Malaria posed a major problem, though. As an eighteen-year-old serving in the U.S. Army Air Corps in the Philippine Islands in 1945–1946, I witnessed the ravages of malaria in the civilian population, especially among children—the shaking chills with temperatures soaring to 105°F, the convulsions, and all too frequently in the younger ones, death.

For optimal protection from malaria, one had to start taking chloroquine two weeks before exposure. I still had a supply of chloroquine at home, left over from my last medical mission to South America. Even though I was beginning a trifle late, I would be certain to pop the first of the chloroquine pills as soon as I arrived home. While in Lagos, I would simply have to rely on insect repellents, a mosquito net, and periodic fogging of my sleeping quarters with Raid House and Garden to keep the mosquitoes at bay.

I drove up the curved driveway leading to our two-year-old ranch house.

As I entered the house, I called out in a loud voice that could be heard in Beth's distant bedroom, "I'm home, Beth. Don't get up. I'll be in to see you in a minute or so." Just then the phone rang, and I stepped up to the kitchen counter to pick up the receiver.

It was Peterson's secretary, Dee, calling with the flight schedules. The best flight to London with connections to Lagos was TWA flight 770 that was departing from Chicago's O'Hare International Airport at 7:30 that night and arriving in London at 9:30 tomorrow morning. Dee told me that they were also forwarding this information to Vic Thomas and that the company helicopter would take me to O'Hare. Dee told me they were preparing the document I would need to take with me to the embassy stating that the emergency in Lagos required my expedited visit. They were getting me some traveler's checks hand-carried to my bank, and also had some of the same insecticides and repellents that I used in Argentina packaged and ready for me to pickup at my two o'clock meeting with Peterson.

I thanked Dee for being the chief of command for this venture and told her I would keep her informed about what I was doing and what else I might need. I was again haunted by the thought that I would be arriving in Lagos three or four days after the explosion. If the care of the seriously burned in the local hospitals hadn't been superb, I could feasibly end up counting dead bodies instead of treating patients.

Dee wished me a good trip. Thankfully, Dee was able to handle emergency situations adroitly. She arrived at work each day with a smile and a dedication to help those in need of medical care—and today was no exception.

The door leading from the attached garage to our kitchen burst open, and Mary rushed in. At fifty-three, she was a beautiful slim brunette with a scattering of graying strands of hair. I wheeled around, but before I could welcome her, she anxiously declared, "Beth had me paged at the grocery store. She said that you told her that you were going to Nigeria."

"Yep, I'm on my way." We embraced, and I told her why the sudden trip to Lagos.

"To take care of burned employees?" Her beautiful eyes widened.

"Yes, they want me to evaluate the medical situation. I'm booked on an early-evening TWA flight out of O'Hare to London, then on to Lagos. I could sure use your help in packing for the tropics. It's possibly as hot and humid in

Lagos as it was in the lowlands of Bolivia." I remember giving Mary a quick kiss as Beth made her way into the kitchen using only one of her crutches and holding a large book in her other hand.

"It's the rainy season in Nigeria, Dad," Beth announced. "I just finished reading about it in our encyclopedia." I knew she had been in our library, a large room next to the family room where we housed hundreds of books. In addition to those for medical research and a variety of encyclopedias, I had amassed a large literary collection over the seventeen years I spent earning my PhD in English literature after medical school.

"Thanks for the info, Beth," I replied, giving her my most appreciative smile.

"Boy, Dad, you are really in for it," she continued. "It says here that in Lagos the heaviest rainy period is May through July when both the temperature and humidity are highest. The rain will just make the tropical heat and humidity more unbearable." Tactfully she offered me the encyclopedia, telling me it might be a good time to learn a little more about the country I was about to visit.

Mary stepped in front of me and, looking directly into my eyes, said, "Why don't you take someone along who knows all about burns?"

Her remark smarted. "I know about burns," I replied defensively and headed for the bedroom. I knew she was right and could only hope that Irv would agree to join me on this mission.

Mary followed right behind me. "I remember those burned Dow Chemical workers you helped care for—most died, remember?"

As I pulled open the drawer housing my summer shorts and all-cotton T-shirts, I responded, "Most were caught in a styrene explosion that caused 100 percent total body burns. There was less than one chance in a million that anyone could survive that severe a burn."

I pondered Mary's disturbing comments about the Dow Chemical disasters, and the nightmarish images of dying workers resurfaced. What if the majority of the burns in Nigeria were severe—say, 50 percent total body burns in a dozen or so people? That would present a catastrophic challenge, even in the best of medical facilities. Taking a burn consultant along wasn't just a good idea—it was a critical necessity.

As she followed me into the bedroom, Mary suggested I take Irv with me. I looked back over my shoulder and told her that, as usual, her suggestion was right on target and that I had already left him a message. My hope was that even if he could not accompany me personally, he might be willing to suggest someone who could make the trip—or a burn specialist already located in Nigeria.

As I started sorting through my clothes and packing my suitcase, I told Mary that I was worried about Irv making the trip only to find that no one has been seriously burned and that those who had minor, nonthreatening burns were being well treated.

"Then he simply flies straight back to Ann Arbor," she said nonchalantly. "But if a lot of people are badly burned, he could show the Nigerian doctors the latest and most successful techniques for saving lives, and that would be worth the risk of flying there."

I slipped two white clinic coats into my hang-up bag. Mary was right. Irv was the specialist, and I would need his help no matter what.

Ten minutes later, with my packing finished, I was scanning the article on Nigeria in the encyclopedia when the phone rang. To my delight, it was Irv.

"This is Dr. Feller returning Dr. Stewart's call."

"Irv, you old son of a gun. It's great to hear your voice. It's been a long time."

"Dick, old buddy. It's good to hear your voice again too. It brings back a host of good memories—like that Sunday midnight you and I had to care for that fulminating case of diarrhea."

"You were the one who knew best what to do. I was only a medical student. As I recall, you were a first-year surgical resident and the chief of command."

"And you were the one who had to carry all of the bedpans." A long laugh followed. "Now what can I do for you this time?"

"I need your help."

"Cynthia told me about the burned Nigerians."

I quickly outlined the events of the day and explained that because of the poor communications, I didn't know how serious any of the burns were or how well the Johnson employees were being cared for.

"All the burned patients are Nigerians?" he queried. "No Americans involved?"

"That's correct."

"And the parent company for this Nigerian subsidiary is American?"

"Yes. SC Johnson and Son."

"Never heard of it."

"Some still refer to it as Johnson Wax—a special wax that SC Johnson introduced that launched the company." I paused momentarily. "It's a big company, Irv—a multibillion-dollar operation."

"And you are the corporate medical director?"

"Yes, but I'm only responsible for the U.S. companies, not those overseas."

"But you have been asked to check on thirty or so burn patients in Nigeria?"

"Yes."

"This could pose a big problem. There are no burn centers in all Africa."

I paused, shocked. This was news to me. I wondered if I could get permission to have Irv join me on this trip to Nigeria. Perhaps the company would pay his way over and offer a consultation fee. "Irv, if I can get clearance will you come with me? I could surely use your help."

Irv was still an adventurer at heart, and I knew that he was a member of the Explorers Club. I hoped he hadn't explored much of Africa on his yearly world expeditions and that Nigeria might be the bait I needed to snare him.

"You know, Dick, I have always wanted to see the Pyramids," he offhandedly remarked. I was taken aback but let it pass, hoping that he was just joking—or at least that he wouldn't bring up the Pyramids again before we were on the plane.

"If I get the go ahead, can you meet me at O'Hare tonight in the TWA lounge by at least 5:30?" I winced, almost certain that I was about to receive a polite "no."

"That could be a bit tight, but I believe I can make it. And before you ask, I do have a passport, but no visa if one is required." A wave of relief like I've never known before flooded over me. If Irv was on board, things were finally starting to fall into place.

"Great! Thank you. I'll call you back as soon as I can with everything in hand—tickets, traveler's checks, signed visa applications, emergency rations, insect repellents—everything except for your toothbrush and clothing. Clothing is important. Nigeria is enjoying tropical weather in their rainy season this time of the year. And don't forget your stethoscope." Our conversation came to an abrupt end when I heard someone in the OR paging Irv.

I first met Irv Feller in 1954 when I was a medical student and he was a surgical resident at the University of Michigan Medical Center. Even then he had the reputation for being a maverick entrepreneur, constantly looking for new ways to improve medical care.

During Irv's second year as a resident, he was assigned to pediatric surgery; and for the first time in his career, he cared for patients younger than fifteen, and he became obsessed with finding a better way to treat skin burns after the admission of two patients with body burns. One day a little boy and a little girl, ages seven and eight, were admitted to the hospital. The boy had a small burn on his leg and the girl a smaller burn on her side. After two weeks of routine treatment, both suddenly died. Irv had kids of his own by this point, and he found this terribly shocking. He didn't understand why the two had died so unexpectedly, especially since their burns were so small.

Irv viewed the children's deaths as a new challenge—he wanted to discover precisely why they had died and to determine how to better treat burn patients in general.

He went to the pathology department, and with the help of Dr. Robert Hendrix, a senior pathologist, the two reviewed the records of the 558 burn patients admitted to the hospital between January 1946 and June 1961. Of these, eighty-five had died. Autopsies had been performed on sixty of them, and infection was responsible for the largest number of deaths—thirty-seven of the sixty patients. These infections were not just localized to the burn areas but were widespread throughout the body, damaging all the major organs. There were septic infarcts with abscesses in the heart, lungs, and brain. Of great surprise to Irv was that each of the thirty-seven had gigantic hemorrhagic adrenal glands—three to four times the normal size—believed to be caused by the terrible stress of blood-borne infections. He concluded that both patient hygiene and antibiotic therapy had to be dramatically improved to increase the survival rate for burn victims.

Dr. Feller's first success in improving the survival of seriously burned patients came a few months later. In March 1957, a seven-year-old girl with burns over 70 percent of her body was admitted. Sixty percent of the burned skin was the potentially lethal full-thickness skin burn—a fatal amount. Irv remembered from his previous study of the medical records that no one with a greater than 40 percent total body burn or a 20 percent full-thickness skin burn had ever survived at the University of Michigan hospital. The seven-year-old girl was doomed—unless she received treatment superior to that dictated by the current burn protocols.

Dr. Feller was granted permission to employ several new treatments on the girl since her prognosis was very poor. He removed her to an isolated sterile room to lessen the exposure of her burned and dying skin to hospital germs—a first at the hospital. When the first sign of an infection appeared, he administered what most doctors at the time viewed as a massive overdose of antibiotics—amounts that are actually standard use today. To care for his patient twenty-four hours a day without interruption, he assembled a select burn care team to cover all facets of treatment—another first. This team consisted of special-duty nurses, a pediatrician, an endocrinologist, a physical therapist, a dietitian, a schoolteacher, and a social worker.

Eleven hours after the burn injury, gentle debridement—or removal of the burned tissue—was carried out, and sterile dressings were applied in the operating room. Homografting, the application of donated skin, was necessary for a temporary skin covering until autografting, the application of the patient's own skin from another part of the body, covered the girl's entire burn surface, including her abdomen and thighs. The girl had fourteen operative procedures during six months of hospitalization. To accomplish the large-area debridement followed by skin replacement in the shortest possible time, a team of four surgeons simultaneously performed predetermined portions of each procedure. Using this approach, the surgical team kept the duration of anesthesia for each of the operations to less than three hours.

Irv was obsessed with this case and made the child his private patient during the second month of his rotation. Six months later, he kissed the girl good-bye as she walked out of the hospital. It was this epic medical adventure that prompted Irv to spend the rest of his surgical career establishing a premier burn care center. The girl's life since her survival has been as remarkable as a fairy tale—good education, happy marriage, and two children. And this is why I was so glad Irv was to accompany me to Nigeria. I could only pray that he would work his magic there if need be.

I made a prompt telephone call to inform Bob Peterson that I had invited Dr. Irving Feller, a world-renowned burn expert, to accompany me to Nigeria. He seemed relieved and pleased that the Johnson–Nigeria employees would now be seen by one of the very best burn consultants in the country. Getting the second ticket, money, and help with a second visa wouldn't pose a problem. He would notify Barney Miller in London that now there were two physicians coming and ask him to transport us from the London airport directly to the U.S. Embassy for the visas. Everything would be in place by the time of our two o'clock meeting with Ray Farley.

I drove past the conventional rectangular buildings of downtown Racine on the way to the Johnson Administration Building for my two o'clock meeting with Bob Peterson and Ray Farley. When the curvaceous brick structure and fifteen-story research tower—designed by Frank Lloyd Wright—came into view, I felt the excitement of entering into a sort of fantasy land of design.

The entrance to the SC Johnson facility feels like a ballroom flooded with light. The massive translucent plastic ceiling is supported by sixty hollow reinforced-concrete mushroom-like columns. From a base only nine inches in diameter, each column widens as it ascends two to three stories to support gigantic circular concrete "lily-pad" tops, each twenty feet in diameter, and each supporting sixty tons of weight.

The executives are housed in posh offices located on the third floor, on a mezzanine overlooking the main work stations on the first floor. The entire complex and working environment is a good reflection of the company's business philosophy—a philosophy that I did not fully appreciate until the Nigerian disaster struck.

That the Johnson company had elected to build such an ultramodern structure is worth noting. In 1928, at the age of twenty-eight, Herbert Johnson—Sam's father and the grandson of the founder—became president. The following year, the United States entered the Great Depression, and the company's profits plummeted from $5 million to $3 million. Unlike most employers, Herbert Johnson refused to lay off any employees and instead urged his research staff to focus their efforts on developing superior new products for the home. The first major success occurred in 1932 when they introduced a new self-polishing floor wax called Glo-Coat. Two months from the day of production, half a million pints of Glo-Coat were in stores across the country. A vigorous marketing campaign sent sales skyrocketing, and Glo-Coat became a nationwide success. The business prospered, and Johnson hired more workers. In 1936, a larger administration building for the now-overcrowded Racine plant was desperately needed, and Herbert Johnson hired the esteemed architect Frank Lloyd Wright to design one.

Herbert shared his father's and grandfather's attitudes toward employees with Wright, telling him that when people receive proper wages and proper working conditions, they did not need to organize to fight for what they wanted.

Wright responded with his ingenious design—a large ballroom-like hall that he proclaimed to be as inspiring to live and work in as any cathedral was to worship in.

Can We Get the Help We Need? Racine—Tuesday, 10:15 AM

Construction of the administration building was completed in 1937, and the attached fifteen-story research tower was added in the 1940s.

I took the translucent cylindrical elevator to the mezzanine and approached the entrance to Ray Farley's office. Ray and Bob were standing just inside, engaged in animated conversation. I suspected they were discussing the astronomical costs the parent company would incur if it decided to fund the prolonged hospitalizations and plastic surgeries for the severely burned Nigerians. If twenty or more employees had 30 to 50 percent total body burns, the cost could very well spiral to several millions of dollars, an amount no small subsidiary could possibly afford. I later discovered this was not the topic of their conversation and that money was not even on their minds at the time.

Ray turned and welcomed me with a warm handshake and told me he was glad I had agreed to go to Nigeria on such short notice. He smiled and told me he was pleased that I was taking a burn expert with me.

Ray motioned for the three of us to be seated at the small oval conference table at the far end of his office. Gesturing toward the coffee machine, he asked if we'd like a cup, and then we began our meeting.

I lifted my coffee mug and took several sips. We briefly talked about the possible need for medical supplies and additional help, and then I stood up, commenting that I had a lot to accomplish before rushing to the airport. Ray and Bob wished me good luck, and I left through the magnificent lobby, praying that Irv's and my mission would not be in vain.

CHAPTER 4

We're on the Way: O'Hare International Airport, Chicago—Tuesday, 6:00 PM

When I arrived at O'Hare International Airport, Irv was waiting for me. At fifty-seven, he moved with the grace of a much younger man. Only the neatly trimmed gray hair and a few wrinkles revealed his true age. He was casually dressed and greeted me with a broad smile. I breathed a sigh of relief, recognizing that he was, indeed, eagerly looking forward to our upcoming challenges in Nigeria. I set my two bags down and reached out to shake his hand.

"Irv, it's good to see you again. It's been awhile since we took care of a patient together. Thank you, again, for coming along," I said, gripping the hand of one of the cleverest surgeons I have ever met.

"No problem, my friend. I've always wanted to visit Africa." He paused a moment, and I prayed he wouldn't mention the Pyramids again. "Although given a choice," he commented, "I wouldn't have picked Nigeria in the middle of its tropical summer."

I handed Irv his tickets, his visa application, and a copy of the letter Bob Peterson wrote in support of the application. Then I reached down and picked up my bags. "Let's check in now so we can relax for a few minutes in the lounge." Ten minutes later, we were comfortably seated and sipping Cokes and briefing each other on what had transpired since our earlier talk—packing tropical clothing, insect repellants, emergency rations, and a few key medical supplies.

"These sodas really hit the spot," Irv remarked, slouching back comfortably in his chair. "It was a long day in surgery—seven kids with hideous burn scars on their eyelids, noses, ears, and cheeks." He turned toward me and asked, "Just what are we in for the next couple of days? We've already missed the time when we could have done the best for any Nigerian with greater than a 10 to 20 percent total body burn." Before I could comment, he sat up straight and asked, "Just who is going to meet us at the airport to speed things up?"

I told Irv that upon our arrival at the London airport, the senior Johnson executive for Africa and the Near East, Barney Miller, would rush us to the American embassy so we could expedite the visa process. Ambassador Louis was also alerted that we were coming, and with the aid of the American embassy, he would make sure our emergency visas were processed and back in our hands by the time we boarded Air Nigeria flight 803 to Lagos.

"Let me get this straight, Dick. Johnson–Nigeria is a small subsidiary of the parent U.S. company, so if the cost of

We're on the Way: O'Hare International Airport, Chicago—Tuesday, 6:00 PM

the medical care exceeds what the subsidiary can afford, then the excess will come out of Sam Johnson's pocketbook?"

I shrugged my shoulders. "I simply don't know how Johnson handles the medical expenses of its foreign subsidiaries. All I know is that they have asked me to advise them as to what best can be done."

Leaning back in his chair, Irv looked at me: "Tell me more about this multinational company, Dick. To be truthful, I never knew it existed until our telephone conversation today. For years I've believed you were working for Johnson & Johnson."

"You're not alone. I had never heard of SC Johnson either until I joined the faculty at the Medical College of Wisconsin in 1966. Then one fine spring day, at my wife's suggestion, we drove the twenty miles to Racine to view SC Johnson's ultramodern administration complex." I explained that Mary was fascinated by Wright's work, and Irv concurred. I described the building in detail, especially the fifteen-story tower. Irv, who was a photography buff, remained rapt in my description of the facility.

Our conversation was abruptly interrupted by the announcement that we should board our flight. We enjoyed our on-flight dinner, and then, taking our nightcaps, we decided to skip the movie and get some much-needed sleep. It was going to be a short night. In less than five hours, we would be landing in London.

I leaned back in my reclined seat and glanced over at Irv. His eyes were already closed. Irv was one interesting fellow, I thought. Since early childhood, his life had been a perpetual struggle, but he always viewed each of the challenges as another adventure.

In 1912, at age twelve or thirteen, Irv's father immigrated to the United States from a small village in Poland. His father manufactured jewelry in New York City and then moved to Upstate New York, where Irv was born in 1925. Irv was an avid photographer, but after high school, he attended a two-year agricultural school in Farmingdale, on Long Island. To cover his school expenses, he worked as a waiter during the day and as an assistant to a veterinarian after school.

When Irv was drafted in 1943, his camera came with him, along with a small supply of Kodak 120 film. During the war, he photographed the camps and surrounding areas, mailing pictures back home. While with the combat engineers, he was assigned to managing the pharmacy, and in his spare time he set up a darkroom and became the unit's unofficial photographer. In December 1944, the unit was sent to Europe, and Irv's commander gave him permission to continue his hobby. He photographed key scenes in England, France, Belgium, and Germany, taking additional photos of his comrades in arms. When Germany was liberated, Irv was given permission to retrace the unit's path through Germany and Belgium, photographing all the destroyed bridges the unit had repaired and the new ones it had built.

Returning home in 1946, Irv promptly began his premedical studies at the City College of New York. Determined to become a physician with a specialty in surgery, he paid for his undergraduate degree by working for a jewelry company.

Irv's speech professor, William Austin, had attended the University of Michigan and, learning that Irv wanted to become a doctor, told him that if he hated a long commute, he should consider the University of Michigan Medical

School, which boasted one of the best surgeons in the world—Dr. Frederick Coller. Professor Austin suggested that Irv take some courses at Michigan and try out the campus. In the summer of '48, Irv did just that, and decided the University of Michigan Medical School was where he wanted to train.

In 1949, Irv was one of several thousand applicants vying for one the 150–200 freshman seats at the University of Michigan Medical School. He was devastated when his application was rejected, which he later learned was due to the quota for Jewish students set in place at the time. The assistant dean of the medical school encouraged Irv to wait a year and reapply, at which time he would be admitted. So Irv spent a year working in the laboratory of Dr. Kahn (of syphilis serology test fame).

Irv entered medical school in 1950, using the GI Bill to pay for tuition, books, and a small stipend. He proved to be a wizard in anatomy, and the chairman of anatomy asked that he teach anatomy to dental students in the following years. This salary was an income godsend, and he taught this anatomy course for the next three years. "It was great for me," he confessed when I was a senior medical student. "You really get to know a subject when you teach it."

Irv graduated from medical school in 1954, and his experience as a surgical scrub nurse at St. Joseph's Hospital solidified his passion toward being a surgeon, a path he never veered from.

I peeked out at Irv one last time. He was fast asleep. I closed my eyes and drifted off to sleep, suspecting that he had a camera and film tucked away in his baggage. This unique physician was still an entrepreneur who embraced life and lived it to the hilt.

We were awakened from our short slumber four hours later when the overhead cabin lights were turned on. I stretched and glanced about. Smiling flight attendants were serving a fine breakfast of orange juice, hot biscuits, real scrambled eggs, strips of hot bacon, a side order of pancakes smothered in syrup, and steaming black coffee. A few of the passengers waved the stewardesses off, closed their eyes, and returned to sleep. Irv and I sat up and relished every morsel of the delicious fare, knowing that it could well be a few days before we would enjoy another hearty American meal.

CHAPTER 5

We Have a Bit of a Problem, Gentlemen: London— Wednesday, 9:05 AM

At 9:00 AM—3:00 AM Wisconsin time—we landed at London's Heathrow Airport, made our way through immigration and customs, and were met by Barney Miller as we left baggage claim. As Barney hurried us to his car in the parking structure, I noticed that the demeanor of this fifty-three-year-old gentleman was decidedly different than when I first met him on a Mediterranean cruise shortly after I began consulting for SC Johnson. Today, Miller's jocular attitude, comedic tendencies, and infectious smile were all absent.

Ten years ago, in September 1972, my wife Mary and I had been invited to attend SC Johnson's global conference in Greece aboard a luxurious cruise ship, the *Aquarius*, along with four hundred Johnson attendees from around the world. At the time, I was a professor of internal medicine and chairman of the Department of Environmental Medicine at the Medical College of Wisconsin.

My "vacation" aboard the *Aquarius* had been hectic—far from the restful cruise my wife and I were promised. By the end of our first three days at sea, one-third of the attendees were ill, many suffering from travelers' diarrhea. Three Australian women were limping painfully on badly swollen legs—a symptom of their long flight—and one of the most influential U.S. bankers had a large boil in his right armpit. The ship's doctor—a Belgian physician—recommended that those with more serious illnesses be dropped off at the closest hospitals on shore.

As I was Johnson's newly hired medical consultant, the attendees felt free to ask me to render a second opinion before the mass exodus to local hospitals began. I made many my "personal" patients while on board, which kept me busy for a few days. Even though I was tending to quite a few people, the cases of diarrhea continued to increase, and I soon discovered that most people simply had not been warned about the dangers of consuming water and snacks from venders on shore in Greece.

With Sam Johnson's permission, I went on the early-morning intercom announcement program and gave the attendees a crash course in eating and drinking safely in Greece, the prevention of overexposure to the sun, and the necessity for protection against mosquitoes. I repeated this information each morning for the next two days. After four days, things were improving, so I stepped down as the morning tutor—only to be replaced by Barney Miller.

"Good morning! Good morning! This is Dr. Stewart," Barney Miller's voice blurted out, much to my mortification.

We Have a Bit of a Problem, Gentlemen: London— Wednesday, 9:05 AM

"Now listen carefully, all of you, and do precisely as I say. Don't drink the water! Don't eat the food! Slap every mosquito! And stay out of the sun! This is Dr. Stewart signing off and wishing each of you a great day!"

I angrily strode into the dining hall for breakfast to search out and verbally whiplash Barney. As I looked about for the culprit, I heard from others in the hall that Barney was considered the company comedian, and also a great musician. Eventually, I ran into him; and with a big grin on his face, he apologized for any hard feeling due to his broadcast. This started the beginning of our lasting friendship.

I learned that Barney was born in Los Angeles in 1929, but after his parents' divorce and his mother's remarriage to an Englishman named Alf Roberts, who was developing a paint-manufacturing business in Buenos Aires, he moved there and developed into a multitalented individual. While in college, Barney became a competitive runner and swimmer. At the age of eighteen, he broke the school one-mile track record while running barefoot on a cinder track. He also loved theater and performed in musicals. Barney went to Cambridge to study for his advanced degree in history—and to continue pursuing his passion for swimming and the theater. He was the swimming champion in the 220-yard freestyle and a regular performer in the annual cabaret show.

It was in England where Barney met his wife, Diana; and the couple moved back to Argentina to raise their four children and Barney worked as an executive in his stepfather's paint-manufacturing business. When that business was acquired by SC Johnson, Alf and Barney became executives with the parent company.

The seriousness of the situation in Nigeria had obviously made a grave impact on Barney. As the senior Johnson executive in the region, he had assumed the role of a general who now had the responsibility of caring for his badly injured troops. Barney quickly placed our bags in the trunk of his car and motioned for us to be seated. I took the passenger seat to his left while Irv scrambled into the roomier rear compartment.

"We have a bit of a problem, gentlemen," Barney apologized as we exited the airport. "An unavoidable traffic snarl due to a tube strike. It's terrible—bumper to bumper and moving at a snail's pace. Sorry about this delay, but Lady Luck isn't in our corner just now."

For the first time ever, I was witness to Barney's serious, businessman side—a side of his personality that I could only imagine had rapidly elevated him to his current executive post, responsible for Saudi Arabia, Iraq, Iran, Cyprus, Egypt, Kenya, South Africa, Nigeria, and Ghana. Miller concentrated on the busy drive from the airport to the embassy, a drive that normally took thirty to forty minutes but stretched to an hour and a half with the congestion.

Irv broke the silence by leaning forward and resting his hands on the back of the two front seats, asking, "Tell me, Barney, have any of the Nigerian physicians suggested flying the more severely burned employees to one of the burn centers in Europe?" He paused a moment, then commented, "As you may know, there are none in all of Africa."

Keeping his eyes focused on the slow-moving traffic, Barney commented, "Taking the Nigerians to a genuine burn center in Europe is a novel idea. No one has suggested this to me." Shaking his head as he viewed the long line of vehicles crawling along in front of us, he remarked, "All I do know is that the majority of the more seriously burned are expected to die."

I glanced back at Irv. I could tell by the serious expression on his face that he was adding up the critical lost hours and calculating the odds against the survival of any of the severely burned who were not receiving optimal care.

We finally arrived at the American embassy, an impressive multistory structure, shortly before noon, and the three of us hurried inside to meet with Ambassador John Jeffry Louis, Jr. We were first taken to meet with Deputy Chief Edward Streator, who had been expecting us. He arranged for a vice consul to rush our passports and necessary applications over to the Nigerian embassy to obtain the required visas. Then he ushered us into the ambassador's spacious office. The ambassador, a tall man around my age, stepped out from behind his desk to greet us. He nodded to Barney and told me it was good to see me again but that he was sorry it had to be under such unfavorable conditions.

I had had the pleasure of meeting Ambassador Louis on two previous occasions at the Johnson global conferences. He served as a member of the Johnson board of directors, and though I had never had a formal meeting with him, I was glad to be introducing Irv to such a fascinating entrepreneur.

Born in Winnetka, Illinois, Ambassador Louis—Sam Johnson's first cousin—had enlisted in the U.S. Army Air Force during World War II, qualifying for cadet pilot training. Following his discharge, he earned his BA from Williams College and an MBA from Dartmouth. From 1958 to1961, he served as the director of international marketing at SC Johnson and then became chairman of the board of

KTAR broadcasting company, which he merged with the Gannett Company Inc.—then the largest newspaper chain in the United States—creating the Combined Communication Corporation. In 1972, he was appointed special ambassador to the Republic of Gabon (West Africa), representing President Nixon at the country's twelfth Anniversary of Independence. In 1981, he accepted placement as American ambassador to the U.K. and Northern Ireland.

As we sat down in his office, Ambassador Louis glanced at his watch and told us our passports would be delivered to us early that evening at the Hotel Excelsior by the driver who would be transporting us to the airport. He said he had notified the American embassy in Lagos of our arrival, and they had agreed to provide us with whatever we needed—medicines, telephone communication, and so forth. He said they ran a good show and we should trust them and use them. The ambassador smiled for the first time and suggested that we check into our hotel and use the free afternoon to catch up on sleep—and do any last-minute shopping for supplies we may need.

The meeting with the ambassador concluded, we stood and shook hands as he wished us well.

On the short drive to the Excelsior, then a luxury hotel, I glanced at the list of items we still needed. At the top was Paludrine, the preventive medication that the Europeans used to protect themselves from malaria, a medicine not available in the United States because it lacked approval by the Food and Drug Administration. With two Paludrine tablets each day, one had good malaria protection within eighteen to twenty-four hours in contrast to the two-week delay with the chloroquine, which I had hastily taken before leaving the States. The second item on the list was a hearty supply of candy bars, a safe substitute for any local food we could not eat.

When Barney dropped us off at the hotel, he gave me some British currency and promised to get us a supply of Paludrine. With the money, I purchased an extra film for my Nikon camera, backup batteries, a hefty supply of Baby Ruth and Nestle chocolate bars, and a small carrying case for Irv. Then we both enjoyed a short nap.

At 7:00 PM, a driver arrived to take us to the airport for our 9:20 PM departure on Air Nigeria 803. He handed us our passports, visas, and the Paludrine. After one brief stopover, our flight was scheduled to land at Lagos at 5:41 the next morning. However, when we arrived at the gate, we were informed that our flight was delayed for an indefinite period of time. Fortunately, there was a lounge where we could chat and sip some American sodas. Finally, at 11:00 PM, we were ushered aboard for a midnight takeoff. Another three hours were lost—precious hours that probably could cost more Nigerian lives.

After the plane reached cruising altitude, I closed my eyes and relaxed. As I drifted off to sleep, scenes of my previous experiences with burn patients materialized and paraded one by one across the stage of my memory. The stage darkened when I vividly relived the moment in the early 1960s at the bedside of a severely burned forty-year-old Dow Chemical technician. He was semi-comatose and lay before me dying. Our team of three doctors and four nurses had exhausted every medical option to prevent his demise, but to no avail.

Five days earlier the man had tripped and fallen into a huge cauldron filled with a bubbling-hot acid solution. He was quickly pulled screaming from the cauldron, washed, and decontaminated; but to everyone's horror, second-degree burns covered his entire body. He was transported immediately to an aseptic hospital room where our burn team used the best medical treatments available at that time to care for his badly blistered body. For four days he survived, showing improvement each day. Then on the fifth day his temperature soared, and it was obvious that a life-threatening infection had seized his body.

I experienced a chill when the man gasped and slowly exhaled his last breath. His eyes remained open as if focused on the ceiling, a blank expression on his face. With a sigh, I pronounced him dead and leaned over to gently close his eyelids. I had exited the sterile environment and hurried to the waiting room to speak with his thirty-five-year-old wife, a stay-at-home mother of three. Looking into her anxious eyes, I uttered the most gut-wrenching words any doctor ever has to say: *Your husband has died.* Disbelief instantly replaced the anxiety in her face. Then horror seized her, and she fainted.

The autopsy confirmed what we suspected. A devastating bacterial infection had attacked all the major organs in the man's body. The adrenal glands were huge, and the brain looked as if it had been peppered with a shotgun firing millions of tiny bacteria—bacteria that were resistant to the intravenous antibiotics we had administered. Intact human skin is a magnificent shield against the hordes of bacteria that make a home on its surface. As long as the outer layer of skin remains healthy and intact, the body escapes invasion and injury. The man's deep second-degree burn had opened the floodgates and welcomed the deadly bacterial invasion.

The skin is the largest organ of the body, about two square yards in the adult male. It has two anatomic layers called the *epidermis* and the *dermis*. The epidermis is the very thin protective outer layer while the thicker dermis makes up the bulk of the skin. Together these two layers of skin perform several vital functions. They protect against infection, prevent loss of bodily fluids, control body temperature, act as a receptacle for sensory stimuli, produce vitamin D, and determine cosmetic identity. The severity of a burn is influenced by five main factors, including the size and depth of the burn, the person's age and past medical history, and the location on the body.

I found myself hoping that I wouldn't have to look into the anxious eyes of a Nigerian woman and say, "I'm sorry, madam, but I am the bearer of bad news. Your husband has died."

CHAPTER 6

Arriving at the Scene:
Lagos—Thursday, 9:00 AM

When we disembarked in Lagos, we were met by a wall of heat and humidity that nearly knocked us down. The immigration and customs clerk examining our passports, visas, and immunization cards straightened up and said in a commanding voice that we had not been immunized against cholera or yellow fever and that this was a requirement for entrance into this nation.

Looking directly into his eyes and with as determined an expression on my face as I could muster, I said, "We are American doctors rushed here to care for a medical emergency. Please let us by." As we deliberately brushed by him, I offered a loud "Thank you," expecting an alarm bell or a police whistle to summon an airport marshal to detain us. We picked up our pace, and to our relief, only silence followed us.

On the way to the baggage claim, we were intercepted by John Bennett, the chief consul of the U.S. Embassy in Nigeria, along with Jim Keane, who had been at the plant at the time of the explosion. With them were two Nigerian drivers.

Bennett, an immaculately dressed man of medium height, gave us his business card on which he had written three emergency phone numbers in addition to his home phone number. Shaking our hands, he assured us that he was available twenty-four hours a day to assist us with our mission. We were to feel free to use the reliable telephone service at the embassy, and should we decide to transfer any of the burn victims to a medical facility outside of Nigeria, he would help us obtain the necessary papers to do so.

At that moment, I did not know that it could take days for a Nigerian lacking a valid passport or visa to *exit* Nigeria—a delay for a burn victim that could prove lethal. The parole documents Bennett provided a few minutes later circumvented the time-consuming bureaucracy for the severely burned Nigerians who were still alive, granting them a chance for survival.

After Bennett's departure, Jim Keane stepped forward and shook our hands. He was a tall well-proportioned man wearing immaculately pressed slacks and a short-sleeved open-collar sport shirt appropriate for the tropical weather.

Reaching out to grip and shake my hand he said I would never know how glad he was to greet two U.S. physicians. He turned and reached out to take Irv's hand and introduce himself. He told Irv he was the guy who yelled help and here we two were. He had a list of the burned employees for each of us—a grand total of thirty with burns ranging in size from little ones up to 80 percent. He opened the rear door of the car in which we would ride.

An 80 percent total body burn! This shocked me. That victim must have been fully clothed. When clothing ignites, the severity of the burn is greatly increased, often resulting in a large, deep full-thickness skin burn.

Keane said he had put check marks by the names of the twenty-three most seriously burned Nigerians and the names of their next of kin. Those twenty-three were in the three area hospitals we were to visit first. He paused and reached up with his handkerchief to wipe some of the perspiration from his forehead. He informed us that the Nigerian doctors told him that all twenty-three were definitely in the process of dying and could well be dead by the time we reached them today. Several of them were really bad off, especially Mrs. Ajao, a young secretary with four small children at home. She was at General Hospital, along with seven other burned employees.

Keane sat next to Oguamanam, the driver; Irv and I slipped into the rear seat. Keane turned toward us and told us that Akalona, our other driver, would take our baggage directly to the Graz Hotel and that if we were up for it, we could proceed directly to the three hospitals. We nodded in assent. We had already lost three precious days.

Keane told us the Nigerian doctors were well trained but their facilities left a lot to be desired—and were hot as hell inside. There was only electricity for a few hours each day, so we should not expect any fans and air-conditioning. And there was a terrible bed shortage. He said one of the badly burned was at LUTH—that's short for the Lagos University Teaching Hospital and that he had been lying on a stretcher in their emergency room for a couple of days waiting for a bed to open up. The doctors there told Keane that the supplementary government funds for medicines and supplies had been sharply curtailed for the past two years because of the current oil crisis.

The highway that connected the airport to the capital was an unbelievable jumble of slowly moving automobiles totally ignoring any attention to the traffic lanes. The paint strips on the road designating the separation of lanes were used as a compass and a guideline for additional lanes full of cars and buses to creep along. Eventually we entered a very modern business district, which boasted skyscrapers and many street-level banks, but the traffic congestion was atrocious. Six to seven bumper-to-bumper lanes of automobiles and buses maneuvered at a snail's pace on a main roadway designed for four lanes only. As we inched along, we were told what we were witnessing was an everyday occurrence in Lagos, a metropolis known around the world as the Go-Slow City.

In 1982, Lagos was not only the nation's capital and major international port city, but it was the largest city in all of Africa—the sixth largest in the world with a population of between eight and eleven million people. Located on Nigeria's southwest coast, the city included four good-sized islands in a large lagoon—Lagos, Iddo, Victoria, and Ikoyi. These were connected to its mainland towns by a series of bridges. The government offices and the country's business centers were on Lagos Island while most of the embassies, including the American embassy, were located on Victoria Island.

The city was grossly overpopulated from a housing standpoint—a myriad of makeshift, overcrowded shacks built from wooden planks, scraps of metal, and even cardboard boxes occupied the available spaces between the permanent cement, brick, and stone buildings. Most startling were the clusters of heavily populated shacks located underneath the overhead highways that connected parts of the city.

During a long delay in traffic, I glanced over the list of the thirty burn patients—their unpronounceable Nigerian names, their ages, their positions with Johnson–Nigeria, and for the twenty-three hospitalized patients, their next of kin. Seven of those hospitalized held managerial or research positions—the general manager, as well as the managers of finance, operations, and planning, also the maintenance supervisor, a chemist, and an accounts clerk. What surprised me the most was that fourteen of the thirty victims were so-called casual employees, meaning they were temporary workers rather than permanent staff members. They ranged in ages from their late teens to twenties—and eleven of them had been hospitalized with severe burns. One of them was the only woman on the list, the young mother that Keane seemed so concerned about.

As we drove, Keane told us about the horrible scene he had witnessed as he came down the steps from the general manager's office on the second floor of the plant. He saw the burn victims being helped into automobiles and rushed off to area hospitals.

Keane explained that Allison Ehiemere, the general manager, had been badly burned on his face and arms during the fireball explosion but had still managed to get the other burn victims into cars to take them to hospitals. He then ordered someone to rush him along with several employees to the Ajanaku Hospital. The company had a contractual arrangement with this small hospital for the health care of its employees. He knew that none of the hospitals in Nigeria, including the Ajanaku Hospital and the large Lagos University Teaching Hospital, had the medicines, the IV fluids, or the equipment to care for seriously burned patients. In Nigeria in 1982, a severe burn was an automatic death sentence. To counter the chaotic logjam of Lagos traffic, Allison had deliberately instructed the driver of the car to swerve to the wrong side of the road and drive where there was little traffic. He ordered the assistant driver to perch on the hood and wave his arms to the oncoming cars, yelling, "Accident, accident, accident."

Keane had joined Mr. Fowode to check on the status of the employees. He told us about their visitation to the various hospitals where the victims were being held. The temperatures in the larger hospitals had been well over 90°F and the relative humidity 100 percent.

As Keane related the events following the explosion and his hospital visits, I began to wonder if Johnson–Nigeria would (or could) offer the same costly medical care to its casual workers as it did its permanent and executive employees. As the U.S. medical representative from the parent company, I had been asked to consult on the adequacy of the medical care being received by each of the burn victims and to help supply the medicines that were not available at each hospital. If my recommendations proved too costly, I suspected the casual workers who had been hospitalized might be excluded from treatment. No one had briefed me on how all this would be paid for, I quickly realized. Soon I would see firsthand how the medical care for Johnson–Nigeria employees compared with that of SC Johnson's three thousand U.S. employees—and I was nervous about the outcome.

In 1976, on the one-hundredth anniversary of the company, Sam Johnson had assembled three hundred Johnson delegates from all over the world, including consultants like me, and composed a very detailed code of corporate social responsibility called "This We Believe," based on the basic principles first summarized in 1927 by his father: *Every employee is a valuable member of the Johnson team. Each is respected and will be treated equally.*

While these principles might be applicable for the three thousand U.S. employees, would they be equally applicable in Africa? I wasn't sure. The small Nigerian operation couldn't possibly afford to pay the medical expenses for more than one or two badly burned employees, and the proper care for two dozen or so badly burned Nigerians would cost a small fortune.

CHAPTER 7

No African Hospitals Can Help: Lagos—Thursday, Noon

We drove bumper-to-bumper through the congested streets to LUTH, where five of the Nigerian burn victims were staying. I anticipated that the treatment of the Johnson employees here would be superior to what the other burn patients were receiving elsewhere in the city, as the hospital was judged to be one of the best in all of Africa.

From the exterior, LUTH did look like the typical university hospital; it was an impressive multistoried structure with countless large windows. As we'd been informed, however, the building was situated in a swampy area—the perfect breeding ground for malaria-carrying mosquitoes. (Later, I asked about mosquito control and was told that usually it was not a problem since most adult Nigerians had been infected with malaria in childhood and those who survived remained immune to the diseases, as long as they were bitten and infected again year after year.)

Though the hospital's exterior was impressive, stepping into the main hall was like entering a shadowy cathedral—the only interior light came peeping through the windows. I was shocked that no overhead electrical lights were on. Tall fans positioned in the hallways stood silently motionless. A musty odor permeated the dense air, which was made more obnoxious by the atrociously uncomfortable humidity and temperatures reaching into the nineties. The hot, fetid air made breathing instantaneously uncomfortable—and it was even more of a nightmare for the patients housed within.

Three doctors greeted us in the hallway. The attending physician—a tall older gentleman wearing a calf-length white clinic coat with his name embroidered above the left upper pocket—was accompanied by two younger doctors wearing shorter white coats. The older gentleman introduced himself and the two resident physicians in training, shook our hands, and directed us to follow him to the bedsides of the five burned patients.

As he escorted us through the corridors, we observed that the hospital was certainly overcrowded with patients, many of whom appeared to be in the throes of dying. They lay in beds crowded together in large open wards, each of which housed over twenty patients. We were told that the lack of space precluded private rooms for the critically ill or isolated rooms for seriously burned patients. Patient care was further compromised by daily electricity outages, a persistent problem that had become a part of normal operations for years. Furthermore, the use of backup generators for hours each day was more than their current budget could accommodate.

The first three of the five burned employees were men in their early twenties with burns over 10 to 20 percent of their bodies. Each was conscious and heavily bandaged. The attending physician felt there was a good chance all three would survive if their wounds didn't become infected. The problem was that many of the patients in adjacent beds did have infections and were potentially contagious. With limited available water, the staff carefully washed their wounds each day and applied fresh sterile dressings. At each patient's bedside, the attending physician introduced me and Irv and then engaged in conversation while checking the patient's charts, sharing the patient's stats with us. I noted that each patient smiled at the physician—apparently he had good bedside rapport.

The fourth patient lay bandaged like an Egyptian mummy in another twenty-plus-person ward. A low moan rose from his motionless body. His eyes were partially open, encircled by wrinkled black strips that had once been eyelids. He had burns over 70 percent of his body, the majority of which were full thickness and extremely deep.

The attending physician turned to us and, in a quiet voice, told us that this man was not expected to survive. In Nigeria no one survived bad burns—and no one wished to survive them either. Severe burns leave ugly scars, and this, in turn, would essentially brand a person as a leper—a despised social outcast for life. No one in the community wanted this fate.

The attending physician was familiar with Irv's scientific publications on the treatment of burns and envied the centers in the United States that had the staff and the facilities to properly treat extensive full-thickness body burns. He prayed that in time Nigeria would have the money to follow suit.

The fifth employee, with 54 percent total body burns, lay at the far end of the twenty-bed ward. He was semiconscious and struggling with a temperature of 105°F in a room where the interior temperature had already reached the mid-nineties. He too looked like a heavily bandaged mummy. The attending physician simply commented that they had no way to cool him down and that they lacked the antibiotics, the intravenous fluids, and the laboratory support to identify and treat the life-threatening infection that was stealing his life. I glanced over at Irv, and he returned my glance with a grimace and a shrug of his shoulders.

Noting our silent communication, the doctor motioned for us to step away from the bed. He whispered softly to us that no hospital in all of Africa could save this man's life. He said that if they were to attempt to treat him optimally, they would completely deplete their supply of intravenous fluids and antibiotics that could better be used to save the lives of countless other Nigerians. Shrugging his shoulders, he told us that his was not a wealthy nation like ours.

Irv nodded that he understood the man's anguish. I nodded as well but kept my thoughts to myself. *Because you are the wealthiest nation in all of Africa with well-educated and trained doctors, why do you tolerate such an unjust allotment of billions of dollars generated by your oil reserves?* We thanked the physicians for bringing us up to date on the five patients and rushed off to General Hospital, where eight additional Johnson employees had been taken.

General Hospital was smaller than LUTH but cursed by the same problems—high interior temperatures, no electricity for stretches during the day, crowded wards in which our Johnson–Nigeria victims lay in beds immediately adjacent to patients with bacterial infections. Three had burns in the 15 to 20 percent range that weren't immediately life threatening. The other five had burns that were potentially fatal.

Four of the five employees were men ranging in ages from eighteen to the mid-twenties and had burns over their bodies in the 35 to 80 percent range. Each was receiving intravenous fluids and had been given a small dose of antibiotics. Each had a high fever. A twenty-year-old with 80 percent total body burns, the majority of which appeared to be full thickness, was comatose with a recorded body temperature of 106°F. I doubted he would last until sunset. What aggravated me the most was the fact that if he were being cared for in a legitimate burn center—limited in his exposure to other infectious patients—he might have a fair chance at survival.

The final burn victim we visited at General Hospital was Mrs. Ajao, the only woman who had been burned. Her case will be forever etched in my memory, as she was severely burned and had a temperature of over 105°F. As we approached her bed, we observed that she was heavily bandaged and lay motionless except for her shallow breathing. I assumed she had been heavily sedated. Her eyes were closed, and the small portion of her face that wasn't burned revealed her youthful good looks.

I glanced at the list of burn victims Jim Keane had given us and noted that her husband was listed as the next of kin. I imagined how devastated Mr. Ajao would be when Mr. Fowode visited their home and informed him of his wife's impending demise—it was a situation too close to my own experiences.

Mrs. Ajao's physician, a man in his late thirties, stepped away from the bed and speaking softly told us they were doing all they could for this lady despite the obvious fact that from a medical standpoint, she could not be saved. He understood that her church had established an around-the-clock vigil praying for a miracle.

"You undoubtedly know how best to treat a burn patient," Irv interjected, "so it must be terribly frustrating that you lack the facilities, the medicines, and, most importantly, a well-trained burn team to care for her." The doctor agreed that it was.

"How often have you transported a seriously burned patient to one of the European burn centers?" Irv inquired.

The physician paused a moment and then replied that since he had been practicing in Nigeria her could recall only one occasion when one of the wealthy elite had been flown to Europe, but had died during the flight to London.

Irv assumed a very erect posture, turned, and faced me and the doctor. In a commanding voice, he said, "I agreed to consult in these burn cases and to help in any way I can. With no qualms, I strongly recommend that every Johnson employee with greater than a 10 percent full-thickness burn or a 20 percent total body burn who can't be placed in a clean environment and treated with state-of-the-art medicines, intravenous fluids, and multiple daily wound cleansing by a trained burn team be flown *immediately* to one of the European burn centers."

The staff physician raised his eyebrows and asked us to excuse him, but it was his understanding that Johnson–Nigeria was a small manufacturing firm with only sixty permanent employees. He asked how it could possibly afford the expense of such an undertaking, and that flying twenty or more patients to burn centers would, as we Americans say, "break the bank."

"Right you are!" Irv snapped back. "But it's *my* understanding that SC Johnson wouldn't have sent Dr. Stewart and me here to look over the situation if spending money were a major deterrent." He reached over and placed his hand on my shoulder. "Dr. Stewart has briefed me on the parent American company. Believe it or not"—he smiled—"Dick tells me that Johnson places employee welfare above profits."

Inwardly, I shuddered. I had no idea how much such a transfer and treatment of ten to twenty patients would cost. A person with 50 percent total body burns could be hospitalized for months for multiple skin grafts and plastic surgeries. In the United States, the cost might easily be between $300,000 and $500,000 per person.

Irv shifted his feet and looked down: "We've already lost three precious days—by far the most critical time in the treatment of burn patients. I came here with Dick to help save lives, not to count the dead—so here is what I propose. First, we send every Nigerian who can't be optimally treated here to one of the European burn centers—not one of the major hospitals, but to a genuine burn center, most of which are affiliated with the military."

The attending physician told us that by the time we could complete such an undertaking of obtaining passports, visas, and transportation, we would lose another three days—and most of the seriously burned patients would have died. He said the last two we just visited would be dead within the next twenty-four hours.

"Please excuse us for just a moment, Doctor," Irv politely said. He took me and Jim aside and said in a lowered voice, "Dick, if we continue like this, all we are going to accomplish on this consulting trip is to be on hand to help count the dead. I certainly didn't fly here to attend a mass funeral. Let's quickly check on the remaining patients at the Ajanaku and St. Emmanuel Clinic and Maternity Hospitals and see how many should be flown to a burn center. With the approximate number in hand, you can call the Johnson hierarchy and tell them what needs to be done if they truly want to save lives."

Irv, the clever entrepreneur, was initiating another of his energetic campaigns, and I was being pressed into service—only this time I wouldn't be emptying bedpans. I turned to Jim, who was looking across the aisle at Mrs. Ajao, his face draped in sadness.

"Jim, once we've finished visiting the Ajanaku and St. Emmanuel Clinic and Maternity Hospitals, I'll need to get to the U.S. Embassy immediately. Chief Consul Bennett promised to provide us with telephone communication and to help us obtain the emergency visas if we need them. I can call the hierarchy in Racine and relay Irv's recommendations. If they grant permission, as I hope they will, I'll use the embassy phone system to call the burn centers in England, France, and Germany and request emergency assistance. Then I'll see what can be done to get speedy transportation—the U.S. Air Force might be our best bet. Anyway, with John Bennett's help, I'll do my best to help launch this project."

Irv turned and addressed the attending physician: "With your permission, sir, after Dr. Stewart and I complete visiting the burn patients in the final two hospitals, I'll return and help your staff prepare the patients for transfer—show them how best to wash and cleanse the burn wounds and the antibiotics to use. While I'm doing this, Dr. Stewart will take care of the burn center and transportation arrangements. So if you'll please excuse us, we must hurry on."

Jim broke in and said he would ask Oguamanam to drive us to the embassy as soon as we were ready. Meanwhile, Akaloma would meet us at the Ajanaku Hospital so he would be available to take Irv back to the hospitals to help in preparing the patients for transfer. Time was precious, so we would skip the Nigerian employee at the St. Emanuel Clinic and Maternity Hospital. Jim said he was told that he only had minor burns on his arms and insisted on being treated by his own doctor.

When we arrived at the Ajanaku Hospital—an attractive small facility that was established to care for the financially able upper middle class—I noted on the listing of burn patients that eleven of the thirteen housed here held major posts at Johnson–Nigeria. Ajanaku Hospital was the only one in the area that Johnson had a contract with for their employees' health care, and as I later learned, this was why Allison Ehiemere had asked to be taken here after he helped the other burn victims.

This hospital was immaculately clean and reasonably well equipped for a small hospital. Yet the situation at Ajanaku was also desperate. The forty-two-year-old financial manager with 60 percent total body burns had just died. In the bed next to him, the planning manager, with 34 percent total body burns, most of them full thickness, was also dying. Eight other men ranging in ages from nineteen to forty-seven were definitely at death's door. Only four men—including Allison

Ehiemere (with 21 percent total body burns), Oli One (the operations manager with 28 percent total body burns), and the two casual workers with 20 to 28 percent total body burns—appeared to be receiving adequate antibiotics and intravenous fluids. Apparently, these four had been deemed the most likely survivors. However, Irv felt that although these four had a fair chance for survival, they would be best cared for at a European burn center. Their facial burns and scarred hands would require repeated plastic surgeries best handled by well-trained burn surgeons.

While Irv was examining Allison, a striking woman in traditional Nigerian dress and headgear who was standing at his bedside stepped up to me and, in a hushed voice, asked, "Dr. Stewart, may I please speak with you—about my husband, Allison Ehiemere?"

"Let's step outside into the hallway, madam," I replied with a polite smile, gesturing to Jim that I would be right back. I wondered how the woman knew my name, but more surprising to me at the time was the clear enunciation of her words with no hint of a Nigerian accent. And the manner in which she spoke was what I would have expected from an American film star.

"I'm Margaret Ehiemere, Allison's wife," she began. "I'm begging you to please take my husband to a good hospital. He could die here."

"This is why we are here, Margaret—to assist in providing the optimum care for all the employees."

"Thank God!" she gasped. "Maybe they could go to London? Or to an American military hospital? There are no hospitals in all of Africa that can care for badly burned people."

No African Hospitals Can Help: Lagos—Thursday, Noon

"We'll do our best, Margaret. One of the burn centers in Europe would be ideal."

"Oh, thank you, Doctor." She reached out and gripped my hand.

"I must hurry back inside and assist Dr. Feller," I said, holding the door open for her to reenter the ward. "Your English is impeccable, Margaret. You're not a Nigerian?"

"No, I'm an American, born in South Carolina. I graduated from Wayne State in Detroit and have worked as a science teacher and, currently, am a full-time mother."

Hearing Margaret's story, I realized that Irv and I knew very little about the badly burned employees beyond their names, ages, job titles, the extent of their burns, and next of kin. I was determined to get to know each of the patients as well as possible.

At the end of the day, I appraised our situation. At each of the hospitals, the staff had done a remarkable job of initiating the proper emergency treatments for their patients. They were doing all that they could given the limited supplies and the less-than-ideal situations surrounding each hospital. But the scene remained relatively sinister.

I did some quick arithmetic. Of the burn victims at Ajanaku, one with 60 percent total body burns had died, five were in extremely unstable conditions, and seven were on the verge of death. If Irv could upgrade the current treatment at the hospitals, we would be in a far better position to save some of the patients, especially if we could secure a transfer to a European burn center; otherwise, death would be a certain outcome for most, if not all, of the patients in the Nigerian hospitals. We needed to act quickly.

"Jim, while Dr. Feller is finishing up here, will you please ask your driver to take me to the U.S. Embassy?" I asked in an anxious voice, noticing that Irv was listening and nodding approvingly. "I'll call Racine and relay Irv's recommendations. I'll ask Bob Peterson to look into what can be done to get speedy medical transportation for up to twenty-four badly burned people. Then with the embassy's help, I'll try contacting the U.S. Air Force. The military has planes specifically outfitted to transport critically ill patients."

As it stood, Irv and I had two plans of action. The first was to transport the victims to burn centers in Europe, as this was a closer and more viable solution to the current problem. However, if for some reason we were unable to cooperate and secure placement for the patients in Europe, then our plan B was to transport them to the University of Michigan Trauma Burn Center in Ann Arbor. This was less ideal but was something Irv felt strongly about.

Jim replied with a smile of relief and told us he would join me at the embassy after he arranged ground transportation for Dr. Feller's return to the hospitals to prep the patients for departure. He told us that if we could complete this important mission, he was going to treat the three of us and our wives to the most sumptuous dinner known to mankind.

CHAPTER 8

Can We Get Help from Europe?
Lagos—Thursday Afternoon

Irv spent the rest of Thursday instructing the Nigerian doctors as to how best to prepare the patients for immediate transport. My job would be to go to the U.S. Embassy and call the burn centers in Europe to see which ones could take the Nigerians. Then with the help of the embassy, I was to arrange for the airplane transportation, the IV fluids and medications, plus a medical team of doctors and nurses to care for the burn victims during the flight.

The American embassy was an imposing multistoried structure adjacent to a series of embassies on Victoria Island. At its entrance, a U.S. Marine armed with a rifle stood on guard. I stepped out of the car, walked up to the marine, showed him my passport, and introduced myself. He compared my face to the photo on the passport and said he was told I might be arriving there today. He gestured me toward the entrance. Once inside, I showed my passport again and was greeted with a firm handshake and a friendly smile by John Bennett. He was the chief of the Consular Section.

John Bennett was in his mid-forties and dressed comfortably in business attire designed for the tropics. He maintained a professional demeanor as he led me down a hallway to his office. He inquired about my training and experience as a physician and wanted to know more about SC Johnson.

Bennett said he had been anticipating my visit and asked how he could help. As we sat down in his office I summarized our medical situation: currently twenty-three of the more severely burned Johnson–Nigeria employees were hospitalized in three hospitals, none of which had the medical facilities or a trained burn care team to properly care for them. It was imperative that the severely burned Nigerians be immediately given the proper burn care with debridement, critical intravenous fluids, and antibiotics to fight their life-threatening infections. Once established in a proper burn center, their lives could be saved and the hideous burn scars surgically erased, which would then allow the patients to return to their homes as survivors, not as lepers.

Bennett concurred that this would be the ideal situation, since current medical care available in Nigeria was quite poor due to the dire economic situation in the country. Hospitals, such as LUTH, that used to be quite famous for their care now lacked the resources to provide adequate staff and the essential medical supplies to treat seriously ill and burned patients. Due to these circumstances, the general population now regrettably viewed hospitals as places where people went to die instead of places that could cure their illnesses. The embassy was well aware of this precarious health care situation, and to avoid suboptimal medical care, embassy personnel and family members with a serious illness were rushed to a private hospital in Lagos for initial triage and emergency care before being evacuated by plane to a premier hospital or burn center in England or Germany.

Furthermore, Bennett confided in me that many spouses of seriously burned or hurt employees working for European or American firms in Nigeria were made rather wealthy when paid the standard $5,000, and the bottom line of such companies was hardly affected. Sending an employee to be treated in a foreign burn center was almost never done as it was incredibly expensive and most major corporations looked to bypass this option. I looked at Bennett, probably with a shocked expression, and he asked me who could afford to have twenty or more Nigerians treated in a foreign burn center? He told me that the small Nigerian firm in Lagos could not do it without the help of the parent American company. The little Johnson firm here in Lagos can probably afford the $5,000 per death, he told me, but not burn care in one of the European burn centers. He looked up at the ceiling and then back at me before telling me he was here to help in any way he could but first he needed to know who was going to pay the several million dollars I was proposing to spend. To his knowledge, he told me, no other American or European firm doing business in Africa had ever undertaken such a feat.

Bennett's reference to the several-million-dollar figure jolted me, and I vividly remember my reply: "I was asked to come here as a doctor of medicine to ascertain what could be done to provide the optimum care for the burn victims—not as a business guru worried about the red ink on the bottom line."

Frankly, I had little idea about the total cost of the endeavor we'd proposed. I told the chief consul that I had been authorized to get the best possible care for these patients. Bennett nodded and insisted on joining me for a conference call to Johnson headquarters in Racine to learn if the company would pay the high cost needed to properly treat the critically ill patients.

"Mr. Bennett, I would greatly appreciate your help in making a call to Bob Peterson at Johnson headquarters in Racine so I can report my recommendations and present the available options: to continue the current level of medical care in the ill-equipped Nigerian hospitals for all the employees, to limit the medical costs by flying only the four key company officials to burn centers and keeping the rest in Nigeria, to expend all resources to fly only the permanent employees to burn centers, or, finally, to fly all the victims to burn centers." I paused, sat back in my chair, and studied Bennett's face. "I can only tell the corporate office what is best from a medical standpoint. It's up to them to decide how many lives they can afford to save if money is an issue."

Bennett told me to make the call from the phone on the desk next to me and that he would listen in on the extension on his desk. I was surprised that the call went through without the usual delays. When Bob answered, his friendly voice boosted my morale.

It took several minutes to brief Bob on the status of the twenty-three severely burned employees. I emphasized that most would die if we didn't transport promptly them to one of the burn centers in Europe. I stated that I required Bob's help in obtaining an ambulance plane—preferably a military aircraft—with a medical staff to provide the patients with much-needed care during the flight. The bottom line, I laid out for him, was that we would need to use the plane as a portable emergency burn center, and time was of great importance. Bob asked me what it was going to cost.

"It'll be expensive—probably in the millions," I managed to blurt out. "Skin grafting and the multiple plastic surgeries to remove the hideous scars on the face and hands are expensive." He told me he could not authorize more than half a million dollars but would talk with Ray Farley about it.

I interrupted Bob to inform him of the standard policy of paying $5,000 to the families of those Nigerian employees who were killed in a work-related accident.

Bob was silent for a few seconds, and then I faintly heard him speaking to Ray Farley. As I waited, I wished I had mentioned the Johnson motto of "This we believe," in which every Johnson employee is considered a respected, valuable member of the Johnson family.

Within a minute, Bob was back and told me I had permission and to go for it.

I noted John Bennett nodding his head affirmatively. He covered his receiver with his hand and whispered that this would be a first.

As Bob continued, I realized that he had already planned ahead for a burn-center contingency. He said he would notify Barney Miller in London what we're about and told me Barney would be the backup man to call if we need help with admission to the burn centers or with transportation. Next, he said he would call Edward Streator at the American embassy in London—and Ambassador John Louis, who might be of help in gaining access to the main burn center in England. He said he had already alerted Bill Perry that we might need a military hospital plane, and he was ready to pursue that avenue by going right to Congressman Clement Zablocki, the chairman of the House of Foreign Affairs Committee, and if that didn't work, then to Secretary Caspar Weinberger and the Department of Defense. He paused a moment and told me that if we did this right and worked closely with the U.S. Embassy and their phone system, we might be able to accomplish this rescue evacuation in record time.

I have to admit that I was surprised and delighted—and for the moment proud to be a member of the SC Johnson international team.

The next few hours were hectic and quite frustrating. Our top priority was to locate air transportation, as well as doctors, nurses, and medical supplies, once a burn center agreed to take our patients. I initially did not think this would be a complicated process, as I had my American Medical Association card, which required U.S. military to assist any U.S. physician in the case of an emergency. With card in hand, I sat down at Bennett's desk and dialed the number printed on the card.

After introducing myself and explaining the medical crisis I was in, I was promptly transferred to a U.S. colonel. I summarized our desperate situation and explained the reason we needed to transport the Nigerian patients to a burn center via an airplane staffed with medical personnel and supplies for treating the patients through the duration of the flight.

He asked me how many of the burn victims were American. When I said that none were Americans, he told me that military aircraft are not generally used to transport foreign civilians, especially overseas where other nationalities are involved.

Worried but still hopeful, I responded, "This is an acute emergency," mentally bracing my hands against the door that I sensed he was slamming in my face. He said he appreciated my situation, but before he could act, he would need a formal request in triplicate and that it could take up to seventy-two hours for a response. Another major problem, he explained, was flying to Lagos. Getting permission to overfly Libya would be a major diplomatic hurdle. If permission was denied or delayed, as he anticipated it might well be, they would be forced to fly around the back side of Africa, and that could be very time consuming.

I thanked the colonel for his time. He was, after all, only carrying out his orders. I hung up and asked Mr. Bennett if the embassy could help. He confirmed that what the colonel had told me was correct and suggested that the burn centers in Europe might be able to provide the required transportation. He also reminded me that the International SOS assistance organization provided many of the emergency flights for injured civilians. He didn't know if they had access to large hospital planes but would check.

Immediately after the call, I notified Bob Peterson about the situation and asked him to launch his plan to contact the Department of Defense in order to expedite our need for a large hospital plane. Bob reassured me that he was already in talks with the department and would call me the minute he had any definitive information.

Next on the agenda was contacting the European burn centers. First, I phoned the center in East Grinstead, England, and was politely informed that all their available beds were full because of the ongoing conflict with Argentina in the Falkland Islands. Another route was blocked.

The burn centers in France, Germany, and the Netherlands were also either full or could take only one or two patients at most. I wondered if the primary problem might be an underlying racism because all the burn victims were Africans rather than Europeans or Americans.

I had struck out, and irretrievable patient survival time was slipping away quickly. I anticipated Bob's disappointment when I notified him of Europe's lack of available burn center beds, but to my great relief, he remained upbeat and said he'd be in touch with Barney in London to see if he could persuade the British embassy to help pull some strings and to get our patients into any U.K. burn center.

June 24 was a long, frustrating day, and survival time for the burn patients continued to slip away.

CHAPTER 9

Plan B: Lagos—Thursday Evening

It was strikingly apparent to me that we needed to develop and implement plan B because if the European burn centers wouldn't or couldn't accommodate the majority of the Nigerians, we had no option but to take them to the United States. In this grim poker game of playing for human lives, all was not lost. We still had one ace up our sleeve.

I told Bob that while Dr. Feller and I had been checking on the burn victims during our hospital rounds, he had volunteered to take all the badly burned survivors to the University of Michigan Burn Center should we have a problem with the European burn centers. Currently, the Burn Center was operating at full capacity, but because they periodically held practice drills during the Cold War to learn how best to care for incoming mass casualties, they could accommodate the Nigerians. These mass casualty drills featured swift evacuation of all their in-house burn patients to one of five perimeter hospitals whose select staff members had been personally tutored in burn care at the University of Michigan. Activating the drill would immediately open up the ten to twelve beds in the burn center for the most seriously burned employees and open the adjacent wing of the main university hospital reserved for an overflow of mass casualties.

However, in the present situation, this was a move of last resort. Transporting the Nigerians to Ann Arbor, Michigan, would take twice as long as a transfer to the closer European centers would require, a time expenditure that could cost even more lives.

I told Bob that with his full approval, I would contact Dr. Feller and ask him to call the university, tell them of the disastrous dilemma we were facing, and ask that they prepare for a real-life mass-casualty operation.

Bob told me there was no debating plan B, so I should get going. He had asked Bill Perry to follow up on the request for a military plane to fly the burn victims to Michigan; however, Bill was told by the Department of Defense that the prospect of commandeering such a plane was not promising. Because of this discouraging response, Bill arranged for the Johnson request to be communicated directly to Secretary Weinberger, who was unable to take any calls until the next morning.

Chief Consul Bennett stepped back into the office to inform me that he had contacted the International SOS assistance organization in Geneva. SOS proposed sending a fleet of three Falcon 20s with several Learjets flying in formation to transport the Nigerians to the various burn units in Europe, provided that the burn units notified them in advance how many beds were available. SOS also informed him that it did not have a plane capable of

Plan B: Lagos—Thursday Evening

transporting all the burn patients nonstop from Lagos to the United States. I sensed some pessimism in his voice as he relayed the current status.

Bennett proposed that we try to obtain a signed release from each of the conscious burn patients or from their next of kin, granting permission for their transport to one of the European or U.S. burn centers. Bennett would contact Vic Thomas to oversee this assignment. He would then contact Johnson's legal department and alert them to what was happening and to have them prepare for a possible emergency evacuation of the employees. Once these steps were under way, Bennett would proceed to obtain the emergency passports and visas for entrance into the United States or, if luck would have it, one of the closer European countries for each patient.

I profusely thanked him for his continued assistance. Without the embassy's help, I told him, it would most certainly take us days to cut through all the governmental red tape—time that could very well cost the lives of all the severely burned employees.

By late evening, we were still mired in no-man's-land. So far the European burn centers could take only three patients total, and the Red Cross Burn Center in Geneva, Switzerland, had agreed to take five patients. So we had placement for eight of the remaining twenty-three who had a good chance for survival. We still had no confirmation about using a military plane, and the chances were looking slimmer as the minutes ticked by. The situation remained dire.

In the Graz Hotel coffee shop, Irv and I were seated across from each other at a small table. Irv looked over a cup of coffee and said, "This frustrating scenario is tearing at my gut. With every passing hour, we're watching lives slip slowly through our hands. If only we could have taken the Nigerians to our burn center in Ann Arbor within a day following the explosion, we might have had a good chance of saving them all. These delays are proving to be too costly."

"What stops us from renting a large commercial jet and flying everyone to Ann Arbor?" I queried.

"Nothing at all except that they aren't staffed with trained doctors and nurses, nor are they equipped with the essential medical supplies."

"If we could staff and equip a commercial European jet in record time, it would be worth the nearly herculean effort."

Irv looked at me over the top of his glasses, his forehead wrinkled.

"Once the jet lands here in Lagos," I continued, "we could immediately convert it into a miniature burn center and transport all the patients to its air-conditioned environment. The high temperatures in the hospitals are brutal for burn patients with high body temperatures of their own."

"A commercial jet replete with large water tubs in which to bathe the patients and clean their burn areas? I doubt it, Dick."

"No tubs, Irv. Cleaning the wounds and dressing them properly is something you would have to oversee before we board them."

"And the medications, IVs, and antibiotics?"

"We could fly them in with the plane—and the embassy can help us. Bennett told me that each embassy in Lagos has medical supplies that can be borrowed, the Americans have stockpiled IV solutions, the French have the market on antibiotics, the British have—I don't recall exactly. The embassy physician could oversee all this, and with Bennett's help, we could supply the plane with the needed medicines."

"And just who is going to set this operation into motion?"

"Our best bet is Barney Miller."

Irv continued to frown.

"I'll get a hold of Barney and tell him what we need."

Irv glanced at his watch. "It's after midnight in London."

"I'll wake him up and wish him a cheery 'top of the morning' then."

"This is turning into a gigantic roller-coaster ride. If I had only known . . ."

"Knowing your love of adventure, Irv, you wouldn't have missed it."

"You're right. OK, I'll alert the University of Michigan Burn Center we're coming and have them put our mass-disaster plan into action." He glanced at his watch again. "The next flight out of Lagos to the United States is late tomorrow, so I have time to catch a couple hours' sleep, then greet the dawn by visiting each of the hospitals and having them use their limited water and medical supplies to clean and dress the burns of each patient prior to transfer to the airport on Saturday morning. Boy, there better be a plane with a medical team on board waiting for them."

"Let's go for it, old buddy—kind of reminds me of the good old days."

"And don't forget you are the one carrying all of the bedpans, Dick, and the first one is going to be backbreaking—renting a commercial jet and conning some docs and nurses into boarding it."

Cynthia Feller, Irv's wife, was awakened in the middle of the night by Irv's urgent call instructing her to alert the key personnel at the University of Michigan who could set the disaster protocol into action. He asked that she emphasize the gravity of the situation and that they desperately needed to make room for the twenty-three severely burned Nigerians for admission to the burn center.

Later that same morning, Bill Perry, following up on Bob Peterson's request, contacted Congresswoman Beverly Byron on the House Armed Services Committee, who advised that the request for a military hospital plane be forwarded from the U.S. Embassy in Nigeria to the U.S. State Department.

After making our decision to transfer the burn victims to the United States, Irv and I held an urgent meeting with Jim Keane and Vic Thomas. Seated in the small conference room at the Graz Hotel, designated our "war room," Irv and I outlined our latest plan of action.

Vic Thomas listened intently and remarked that he approved of plan B and would help in any way he could. I found this a bit surprising. I had not anticipated his ready approval of a plan that the small Johnson–Nigeria plant could not possibly afford without corporate help, especially a plan that would set a precedent by transporting a large number of Nigerian employees to a foreign country for medical care not available in Africa. If the man was telling the truth, he obviously wasn't one of those working solely for the bottom line.

CHAPTER 10

Looking for Miracles:
London—Friday, 3:00 AM

It was 3:00 AM in London when I called Barney Miller and gave him an almost-impossible task to complete within the next few hours. Time was running out. All the burn patients were dying. I told him that the frustrating response from the European burn centers now dictated a change in plans, and that to save any of the severely burned Nigerians, we were going to fly them directly to the University of Michigan Burn Center. The biggest problem with this new strategy was the difficulty in immediately obtaining a hospital plane for transport—one large enough to transport all the victims nonstop from Lagos to the airport in Detroit. It appeared that there would be an unacceptably long delay if we were to wait for the U.S. military to supply one. What we needed was a large commercial jet—a DC-10—that we could quickly convert into a miniature intensive care burn center staffed with physicians and nurses trained in emergency medicine.

I heard that there was such a group in Great Britain who engaged in emergency medical evacuations and speculated that Barney's personal physician would probably know how to contact the group. I didn't believe that renting a large commercial jet should pose a major problem. The emergency evacuation physicians would know how best to proceed. I asked if he would be willing to make the necessary arrangements.

I paused, hoping for a quick affirmative response, but Barney remained silent. I certainly realized I was asking for a small miracle and sensed that he was now fully awake, and I was debating whether this former championship swimmer and track star was up to the challenge of diving headfirst into the chilly waters to rescue the remaining Nigerian burn patients. I made a silent prayer that his answer would be positive.

"I'll do my best, Dick, to get the commercial jet, doctors and nurses, and medical supplies."

"Thank you, Barney, and the best of luck—many lives are now in your hands."

Greatly relieved at his response, I thought that if anybody could pull off this miracle, it would be a multitalented man like Barney.

Barney later related to me that after he put down the phone, he put on his bathrobe and sat on the edge of his bed to plan how best to go about renting a large commercial jet, staff it with doctors and nurses, and fly them to Lagos. He said he leaned over, kissed his wife Diana, and asked for her help. He and Diana had stayed up until dawn, making a list of people they could call to ask for help. He started phoning contacts early the next morning. He first tried a friend who directed him to contact the Duty Theatre sister at the Royal Survey County Hospital for more information on an ambulance service called Europe Assistance. When he called, he was referred to Sister Corrine Older (she would later volunteer as a nurse on the rescue team). Through Sister Older, Barney had obtained the phone number of Dr. Richard Fairhurst, Europe Assistance's lead physician.

Barney explained that Dr. Fairhurst instantly agreed to assemble a medical team and to help find suitable aircraft for the venture. Dr. Fairhurst was successful in finally locating a DC-10 operated by Martinair Holland out of Amsterdam. Apparently, Dr. Fairhurst, with the help of the London Executive Aviation, was able to charter a British Air Ferries Vickers Viscount to fly the London medical staff to Amsterdam. Barney called to tell me that, by 11:30 in the morning, everything was in place and that he had successfully telegraph-wired a down payment of £123,500 to assistance operations.

At 1:30 PM, the medical team arrived at the airport in Gatwick toting the medical supplies they needed to convert the DC-10 into a hospital plane: Dr. Fairhurst, Dr. David Wood, Dr. D. Laing, Sister Corrine Older, Sister P. Lees, Sister Hillary Robinson, and a man named Khan, who was a medical technician with nursing skills. The team departed Gatwick at 2:30 PM and arrived in Amsterdam at 3:15 PM. They hurried to the airport medical center for yellow fever vaccinations, a requirement for setting foot in Nigeria.

At 5:30 PM, DC-10 flight MP71 departed Amsterdam headed for Lagos. The flight crew consisted of Captain Barkel, First Officer Verryt, Flight Engineer V. Lunsen, and

Loadmaster Alebes. There were eight flight attendants, none of whom had had any nursing experience. So far, so good.

Meanwhile, at daybreak in Ann Arbor, a University of Michigan Disaster Team headed by Associate Hospital Director Howard J. Peterson went into action. Irv notified the burn center that we had no option but to admit all the Nigerian burn victims to the university facility. He informed the staff that he would be taking the next flight to the United States so he could oversee the admission and treatment of the burn patients once the Nigerians arrived at the Detroit airport aboard a commercial jet. The preparation for the incoming burn victims required the rapid assembly of a large number of doctors, nurses, and technical staff ready to perform their vital roles when the jumbo jet landed at Detroit Metropolitan Airport on Saturday. Director Peterson was comfortable with the protocol that had evolved from the hospital's previous experiences with mass casualties and the periodic mass disaster exercises held in conjunction with the military and the other hospitals in the Ann Arbor area.

To free up seven of the beds in Michigan's ten-bed burn care center, the unit's head nurse, Kathleen Dunlap, expedited the redistribution of seven patients to one of the two auxiliary burn care facilities in nearby hospitals. This opened the doors to the unique, self-contained wing of the main hospital, which featured its own sterile ventilating system, operating suite for incoming patients and skin grafting, a hydrotherapy area, and artificial kidney equipment. The burn care unit's capacity was expanded by sealing off an adjacent corridor and incorporating its rooms into the burn care system. Other ICUs in the hospital were alerted to receive patients if necessary.

The hospitals' two head physicians in Emergency Services and its administrator made the arrangements with the U.S. Air Corps for transporting the patients from the Detroit Metropolitan Airport to the burn center via two large helicopters. The helicopters, commonly known as Jolly Green Giants, were staffed by members of the 501st USAF Search and Rescue Squadron. This multistep procedure would require separate medical-nursing teams at the Detroit airport, at the helicopter landing site, and finally at the burn center.

The burn center at Ann Arbor had made great advances under Irv's direction. Prior to 1959, when he was appointed clinical director of the burn program, there was no formal burn care program available. No single physician was in charge of burn patient care, and most patients with major burns greater than 25 percent died. Under Irv's visionary leadership, though, the University of Michigan Burn Center became the first specialized burn treatment facility in Michigan and one of only a handful in the United States. Initially, the unit had six beds and could accommodate up to one hundred patients each year. The resulting organization of the intensive care management for the burn patients resulted in a dramatic decrease in both mortality and morbidity.

In 1968, a specially designed, self-contained eight-bed unit replaced the original sector at the burn center. To facilitate burn care, it contained its own operating room and a tub room to aid in daily cleaning of patients' burned areas. In that same year, the National Institute for Burn Medicine (NIBM) was founded, and it published a book on burn nursing by

Claudella Archambault Jones, head nurse of the center. It was used by more than eight thousand nurses who were trained in burn care by the educational programs and seminars conducted by NIBM.

And now, thanks in most part to the skillful, rapid help of Barney Miller and his wife Diana, we were ready to take our Nigerian patients to this world-class facility.

CHAPTER 11

Martinair to the Rescue:
Lagos—Saturday, 2:00 AM

The Martinair DC-10 touched down at the Lagos airport shortly before 2:00 AM. The sleepy medical team and aircraft crew were met at the gate by John Bennett and members of the U.S. Embassy, who had arranged with the Nigerian government for transit visas and immigration clearances for them. The bad news was that the DC-10 could not depart until the flight crew had been allowed eight hours of sleep, a union requirement that could not be compromised for any reason.

I was later told that arrangements had been made with the airport officials to allow the medical personnel and aircraft crew easy departure and return. Additional arrangements had also been made to permit the burn patients immediate access to the airport and the use of high-lift loading machines to hoist the stretchers with the patients up to cabin entrance doors.

Flight for Life

Bennett had booked rooms for the air crew and medical staff at the Holiday Inn near the embassy. As he escorted them from the baggage claim area, he explained that, as a precautionary measure, they were proceeding to the hotel in a convoy to avert any potential hijacking, an all-too-frequent occurrence on the road from the airport into Lagos. Just hours earlier, a small bus carrying a four-man German flight crew and eight flight attendants had been hijacked. Armed thugs had blocked the congested airport highway and confiscated at gunpoint everyone's possessions: rings, jewelry, wallets, purses, shoes, and all clothing except for the undergarments. Standing barefooted on the highway, the German crew watched with mouths agape as the hijackers then turned and fled the scene with their loot, triumphantly waving to the line of backed-up motorists.

Bennett led the aircraft crew and medical personnel to his convoy—an American embassy Jeep, two air crew buses, and several automobiles for the medical personnel. The Jeep led the way to the Holiday Inn, with Bennett seated next to the driver—a large fire extinguisher clenched tightly between his knees for immediate use to spray in the face of anyone who attempted to block the road and rob his group. I wondered why Bennett hadn't requested an armed marine to join the convoy but later learned that this show of force would cause any potential hijacker to take more violent measures to overcome the vehicle.

At 2:30 AM, the convoy arrived safely at the hotel, and fifteen minutes later, the medical team and I met to plan for the day ahead of us. Dr. Fairhurst of Europe Assistance introduced me to his team of two physicians and four nurses. Fairhurst and his team nodded knowingly as I described the deplorable situation in the three hospitals.

I explained to Dr. Fairhurst that Vic Thomas would begin transporting the burn victims to the aircraft at daybreak. The onboard air-conditioning would be vastly superior to the 100°F hospital temperatures, especially for the febrile patients, and we could immediately begin the specific intravenous fluid and antibiotic therapies Dr. Feller had requested. In short, the plane's interior would resemble as much as possible a functioning intensive care unit.

Bennett then telephoned me for the latest status of the burn patients. I informed him that I anticipated several more burn victims would die before sunrise and that we would be lucky to have eighteen still breathing when we boarded the plane. He read me the list of medical supplies and equipment on board the DC-10, and I, in turn, detailed the in-flight treatments that Dr. Feller recommended. Obviously, we lacked enough of the antibiotics and intravenous fluids that Dr. Feller felt were so essential, and Bennett promised to deliver the additional medicines directly to the DC-10 prior to our departure.

It was approaching 5:00 AM, and the day's frantic efforts had taken their toll on me. I felt like I was walking in my sleep. I flopped into bed, exhausted. The fatigue reminded me of the twenty-four-hour emergency room ordeals I had experienced years before as a busy University of Michigan Medical School intern at Saginaw General Hospital. I had somehow managed then; I would certainly manage now.

Grateful for two hours of sleep, I staggered to the bathroom and stepped into a lukewarm shower in order to wake up. My eyes wanted to close, so I reached over and turned on a thirty-second blast of icy water. My adrenaline soared! Then I switched back to warm water and with eyes open began to enjoy a quick warm scrub-down. I patted myself dry and managed a smile and a wink at the mirror before I began to shave.

After a quick breakfast—two mugs of steaming black coffee to wash down two hard biscuits—I grabbed my baggage and joined Jim Keane to head to the airport. Low gray clouds threatening to release a torrent of rain darkened the morning sky—the beginning of a day I would never forget. We made excellent time, and the driver dropped us off at the terminal in less than an hour. Inside we were met by Bennett and the embassy's medical officer, who ushered us through immigration and customs and onto the DC-10. Bennett guaranteed that there would be no delay in permitting the burn patients to enter the airport and proceed directly to the plane. He would double-check all the medical supplies and make certain that all the requested items were aboard the DC-10.

As Keane and I stowed our baggage in the first-class compartment, he mentioned something about getting us a delicious Western-style second breakfast on board. I nodded in agreement and walked back to peek into the large economy section. *They did it!* I told myself. *The British medical team had really done it!* A commercial passenger airliner from Holland had been converted into an intensive care unit. Twenty stretchers were securely anchored on top of the passenger seats. Six clotheslines had been strung back and forth between the overhead baggage compartments from which we could conveniently hang the intravenous fluid containers. In the few open seats along the aisles medical equipment had been strategically positioned—four air ambulance kits, four nursing cases, one large case containing Roehampton burn dressings, sixty-five liters of

Martinair to the Rescue: Lagos—Saturday, 2:00 AM

intravenous fluids, six vacuum mattresses, one Paraguard stretcher, over twenty thousand liters of oxygen in cylinders, three electric suction pumps, and even a few defibrillators, which I hoped we would not have to use often.

I glanced out of a rain-splattered side window and looked up at the sky. The low dark clouds had moved on, leaving behind a gray day with drizzling rain. I smiled. Lady Luck had joined us after all. The current weather wouldn't delay our departure once the patients were on board. I noted that there was adequate light inside the plane in order to document our mission with photographs. After all, if this extremely costly mass-rescue attempt succeeded, it would be considered—as John Bennett claimed—a first by any American company in Africa, and it would be beneficial to have it documented. I also planned to dictate a patient-record journal into my handheld tape recorder to preserve the details of the mission.

As I snapped two or three views of the makeshift beds and overhead lines, I grimaced. If only we had had this plane a few days earlier, this rescue would have been far more successful, and we would not now be attempting to tiptoe around a mass graveyard. The eighteen remaining Nigerian burn patients, all of whom had infections for which they had received pitifully inadequate amounts of antibiotics and hydration, as well as poor overall wound care, would hopefully make it to the plane. This was the sixth post-explosion day, and despite our intervention, many could die before we reached the United States.

Keane's high-pitched, excited voice startled me, as he called out for me to look out at the tarmac, that they were coming. My negative thoughts were erased as I turned and looked where he was pointing. Approaching us was a convoy of two small passenger buses led by a black passenger car. The convoy screeched to a halt at our passenger entrance ramp, and two dozen people wearing raincoats stepped out into the drizzle and scampered up the dozen steps entering the plane.

Bennett and the embassy doctor were the first to enter, followed by two embassy employees bringing in the additional medical supplies we deemed essential for optimally treating the burn victims. These extra supplies included sixty million units of penicillin and large boxes filled with IV fluids and burn dressings.

Next, a tall man in his mid-forties held out his hand to me and introduced himself as Captain Barkel of Martinair Holland out of Amsterdam. He said that he and his crew were here to help with the evacuation. Captain Barkel introduced his first officer, flight engineer, and loadmaster. As we exchanged handshakes, the eight flight attendants boarded—attractive young women in bright red uniform jackets and skirts. To my relief the captain and the entire crew spoke fluent English and informed me that while none of the flight attendants had nursing experience, they would be more than happy to help us in any way they could.

When the medical team boarded, I said, "I can't tell you how pleased I am that you have come to help save the lives of the burn patients. Without you and this plane, most would have died." I gestured to the rear of the plane. "The patients should be arriving shortly, so after you hang up your rain gear, let's meet in the passenger compartment that you have so nicely converted into an intensive care unit, and I'll brief you on what I know about the patients." The briefing was interrupted moments later by ten vehicles carrying the Nigerian patients driving across the tarmac toward us. Three white ambulances led the way followed by several vans and four cars. Bringing up the rear was a pickup truck with one patient lying prone on a pile of hay. A decorative Nigerian robe covered his multiple bandages and hospital gown.

I can't believe this, I said to myself, agonizing over the view of a severely burned patient lying on the pile of hay replete with fungi and bacteria. *We're fighting lethal infections so why not invite every type of bacteria in the area to the death party?*

As I scampered down the first-class passenger entrance to oversee the loading of the burn patients, Vic stepped out of one of the cars and waved as he walked briskly toward me.

He greeted me in a surprisingly calm voice and told me he had everything required by immigration and customs in the folder he handed me. He had a list of the eighteen patients that we would be evacuating—two more employees died during the night, so that brought the total of dead to five. Vic—over six feet tall, elegant, and well dressed—handed me a folder with signed copies of the patient and next-of-kin release forms. For a man who must have spent a grueling twenty-four-hours driving around Lagos to the three hospitals and then searching for the homes of the burn victims' wives and their next of kin to persuade them to sign the documents, he certainly looked alert and wide awake. He also told me that four of the burn victims' families wanted their loved ones to remain in the hospitals where they were now and that there was nothing more that we could do about it.

Airport personnel now positioned the high-lift rig directly beneath the passenger doorway and announced that they were ready to begin lifting the stretcher cases up the fifteen to twenty feet to the open doorway. I signaled for the first ambulance to begin the process and watched as they carefully lifted a stretcher bearing a heavily bandaged, apparently unconscious patient and placed it gently on the high-lift rig. All I could see of his badly swollen, charred face were his closed eyes and what looked like a small piece of broken charcoal where his nose had been. He was gasping for air through what was left of his widely parted lips. He appeared terminal—death number six, no doubt.

Damn! If only I had known about the current status of the Nigerian hospitals before I left the United States and could have acted sooner, this man would have had a far better chance of survival. I noted that a name tag was pinned to the front of his hospital gown and check-marked his name on the list of patients that Vic had handed me. I turned to the Nigerian who seemed to be the senior ambulance driver and asked where the patients' hospital records were. The driver told me he had brought the hospital charts that were given to him and that only three of the hospitals sent medical records with him.

This was unbelievable! How were we to know what medications these critically ill patients had received within the past twelve to twenty-four hours? The time and dosage of each of the medicines was crucial information. Worse yet, without the hospital charts, we wouldn't be privy to such essential information as the burn victim's past medical history—the presence of chronic tropical infections, diabetes, or heart disease—information now unavailable if the patient, like this man, was unconscious. We desperately needed the flow sheets showing weight gain or loss since the burn incident, body chemistry measurements, blood pressures, pulse rates, fluid intake, and urine output. *This was turning into the worst nightmare of my medical career.*

And there was another impending problem—the religious beliefs of the various patients. In Nigeria about 47 percent of the population were Muslim, 34 percent Christian, and the rest various other religions. In the Lagos area, 50 percent were Christian and 34 percent Muslim. If this dying man was Muslim, I had no idea of the proper procedure to follow upon his death. When I expressed my concerns, Vic explained the proper burial for all Muslim patients. He stressed that it must be done very smartly and that it was important that they not be buried in the United States. The bodies were to be put on ice and returned to Nigeria.

I glanced upward as the high-lift rig elevated this first patient. Dr. Richard Fairhurst and his crew were now standing in the open doorway, ready to take the stretcher on board. As I raced back and mounted the steps to the first-class entrance, I dictated the spelling of our first patient's name and the time of his admission to our ICU. According to the patient listing, John Akalamna was a twenty-seven-year-old worker with 60 percent total body burns, most of which were reportedly deep third degree. He was semi-comatose and severely dehydrated. Maybe, just maybe, with speedy rehydration we might pull him from the brink of death. As I looked at the suffering man, I could not understand why an oil-rich country, like Nigeria, had such substandard medical facilities and resources for its citizens.

Unable to gain access to a suitable vein in our first patient on board, the British team, without hesitation, administered the critical saline via a rectal enema. Within thirty minutes, John Akalamna regained consciousness and began to ask questions about where he was and where he was being taken and in a loud voice cried out wanting to know if he was dying. He demanded we tell him the truth, asking again if he was dying. Everyone turned to see who was going to answer. I was too far away to hear the reply of the British nurse caring for him, but I did see her lean down and speak to him in quiet whispers. Their conversation continued for several minutes, and when the nurse stepped away to care for another patient, the man appeared calm and relaxed.

I glanced in my folder to see if this man had been conscious and able to sign a consent form. He had, and I noticed that he was single and that his next of kin was an uncle who had also signed a form. John Akalamna—even with so much of his body burned—had a strong desire to live. Because he was the least likely of our patients to survive, I placed him at the top of my priority list.

The second patient brought on board was Dele Jacob, a twenty-eight-year-old accounts clerk—an unmarried man with 53 percent total body burns in his head, neck, arms, hands, trunk, and thighs. As I walked up to his stretcher and looked down at his heavily bandaged body, a foul, slightly nauseating odor enveloped us. His burn wounds needed cleansing, which was going to be difficult during a flight without a clean washtub and a good water supply with which to wash him. Dele looked up at me with wide, frightened eyes on a face that had swollen to the size of a basketball. The burns on his face were positively revolting! If he survived the next week, his facial scarring would be hideous and require weeks of plastic surgeries before he could rejoin society with a smile.

I introduced myself to Dele and told him, "We are taking you to one of the best burn treatment centers in the world, a burn center that will help your body heal and put you back on your feet."

There was a pleading look in his eyes and blurred words coming slowly through swollen, burned lips as he asked if I could get a message to his wife-to-be in Ghana.

"No problem," I assured him. "We can send it via airmail once we land in the United States." Dele blinked his eyes, his swollen, charred eyelids moving slowly, and said thank you.

"Don't try to talk now, just relax," I said, giving him a reassuring smile. He told me he hurt all over. "I know. We will give you the medicines to control the pain and make you feel better." Dele nodded that he understood. I did my best to give him a second reassuring smile and stepped aside to make way for one of the British doctors and a nurse hurrying up the aisle carrying a surgical tray containing the instruments and supplies for performing a surgical incision known as a cutdown. This is a procedure used for patients whose surface veins have been destroyed, in order to gain access to a deeper vein. This way, they were able to administer both life-saving intravenous fluids and antibiotics through Dele's burned skin.

Activity at the passenger entrance doorway caught my attention. The stretchers with two more heavily bandaged patients were being brought aboard—the thirty-seven-year-old operations manager, Oli One, and a twenty-three-year-old factory worker, Okon Bassey. Both had burns on approximately a third of their bodies. Okon was comatose and appeared terminal. There was no accompanying hospital chart to help us determine his most urgent problems. High fever and obvious severe dehydration would dictate immediate intravenous antibiotics and the infusion of fluids. The other patient, Oli One, had been charred on the left side of his face, and his left eyelid, the left ear lobe, and forehead were going to present a major reconstruction task provided we could handle the immediate life-threatening problems—a high temperature indicating sepsis and severe dehydration with possible kidney failure. The accompanying medical records—one of the few we received—confirmed the dehydration problem, recording a dramatic drop in his urine output in the previous twenty-four hours.

I noticed that the feet and ankles of the first four Nigerian patients were burn free. Apparently, they had all had been standing in water when the fiery explosion occurred. Possibly all the remaining fourteen patients would have burn-free feet. If so, my brief medical dictations would be quicker if I referred to each patient by a number rather than fumble with the difficult spelling of their names. I quickly retraced my steps and with a fine-point permanent marker printed a single number on the toenail of each man's great toe. The toenail of John Akalamna became number 1, Dele Jacobs was number 2, Oli One became number 3, Okon Bassey was number 4, and so on.

The sound of two people vomiting cascaded over the soft voices of the doctors and nurses caring for patients in the quietness of the passenger compartment. I glanced quickly at the four patients on board and the next two who were being carried into the plane. None of these were vomiting, but there, in the front of the compartment, two of the flight attendants were doubled over, each retching into one of the small paper vomit bags found in the seatback. This wasn't surprising to me though. The burn victims were as gruesome a group as anyone could imagine. Swollen, blackened skin peeking out around thick white bandages—noses, earlobes, and eyebrows disfigured, charred, or missing and mouths twisted in pain. Heavily bandaged, the patients looked as if they belonged in an old mummy movie—and the foul odor coming from each, though not strong, could be nauseating. I had witnessed first-year medical students not only vomit but also faint when viewing a burned human being for the first time.

Our greatest problem during the flight, though, was that we were shorthanded. To care for eighteen critically injured patients, we ideally needed to double the number of nurses and doctors now assisting us. The extra hands provided by the flight attendants could be lifesaving. I mentally kicked myself for not having thought to inform Barney Miller of the ideal number of medical staff and burn care supplies we would require. As the vomiting continued two other flight attendants hurried down the aisle and stood before me. Their faces were somber and eyes wide, they told me that all of them wanted to help in any way they could, that I should just tell them what to do.

"Thank you, ladies. Your help is desperately needed as you can well imagine. I'll ask the British head nurse to supervise you." I felt that two angels were standing in front of me, and I said, "God bless you."

Patient number 5 was a twenty-one-year-old named Lambert Okpara with 65 percent total body burns. He was conscious, battling a high fever that was complicated by fluid building up in his lungs, a deadly condition known as pulmonary edema. His blood pressure indicated he was in shock, and his pulse rate was far too slow to support his life for long. Even with the best treatment we could offer, it was doubtful he would still be alive upon arrival in

Michigan. Dada Badu, patient number 6, was a twenty-one-year-old with 65 percent largely full-thickness skin burns. Infection had set in, but the harbinger of death included pneumonia in both lungs, kidney failure, severe dehydration, and a sky-high blood sugar.

Patient number 7 was Allison Ehiemere, the company's general manager, a forty-one-year-old with 22 percent of his body burned; he was the least severely burned of the group. Number 8 was Hycenth Munonyi, a thirty-year-old operator with 37 percent of his body burned. Both men were fully conscious, but both appeared dehydrated and had low-grade fevers. Nevertheless, they were harboring bacteria that had the potential to invade the body and kill. With the appropriate antibiotics and fluid therapy, I decided we should be able to stabilize these two. I started their IVs and began their fluid therapy.

Numbers 9 and 10 were questionable survivors. Number 9, Paul Oquamanam, was a twenty-year-old casual worker with 45 percent total body burns, a high fever, and dehydration. Number 10, K. K. Olamayin, a twenty-five-year-old operator, had over 64 percent total body burns, most of them full thickness. His entire head was a swollen, speckled black disaster zone. Both eyes were badly infected, and he was in shock.

Numbers 11 and 12 were also questionable survivors. Number 11, Oyebanji Adekola, was a twenty-one-year-old with 45 percent total body burns and bilateral pneumonia. Number 12, Sibastian Onyensa, was another casual worker, a twenty-two-year-old with 55 percent total body burns, aspiration pneumonia, and bleeding from his gastrointestinal tract. In both patients, high fever, dehydration, and kidney failure were critical challenges to overcome.

The next four patients all had high fevers, were dehydrated, and in dire danger of kidney failure. Number 13, Emmanuel Adeeko, was a forty-seven-year-old with 54 percent body burns; number 14, Michael Enu, twenty-two, was a machine operator with 54 percent total body burns; number 15, Lawrence, a twenty-two-year-old casual worker, had 35 percent total body burns; and number 16, Sule Oduwaye, a forty-one-year-old, had 40 percent total body burns. I looked for Mrs. Ajao, the casual secretary with four young children at home, the lady Jim Keane was so concerned about, but was told that she had not survived.

As the patients were carefully placed on the stretchers, Dr. Fairhurst and his medical team calmly and efficiently accomplished the herculean tasks of beginning the essential lifesaving measures—battling the systemic infections, the high fevers, the severe dehydration, the shock, and the kidney failure that were threatening the lives of the majority of the patients. In record time, they performed eight surgical cut-downs to reach the veins of the patients whose surface veins had been destroyed or were clotted, and administered one liter of saline along with two million units of penicillin that Dr. Feller had recommended they each be given once on board.

To my relief, the two nauseous flight attendants had recovered, and they joined us in helping the severely dehydrated, conscious patients drink copious amounts of fruit juice and water. Their smiles and the encouraging face-to-face conversations they had while holding the straws of juice-filled glasses to the mouths of the weakened patients with heavily bandaged hands had a wondrous effect on the morale of the burn victims.

I kept looking at my watch, anxious for our plane to depart, but the ambulance transporting the last two patients had yet to arrive. It was now 12:30 PM, and the van was nearly an hour late. All that we knew was that it had reportedly left the hospital on time.

To add to the tension, I noted that the weather was worsening. The low-lying clouds had returned, intensifying the rain and enveloping the airport in a dusky gray light. I prayed that the deteriorating weather conditions wouldn't delay our departure once the last two patients were boarded. The minutes we were losing were precious and could be costly.

CHAPTER 12

More Delays: Lagos—Saturday, Noon

While we nervously awaited the two late arrivals, we allowed the wives and next of kin of the burn victims to board the plane and stand beside the stretchers holding their loved ones. It was quite a scene. Wives with tear-streaked cheeks tried their best to smile down at heavily bandaged husbands while bottles of intravenous saline delivering the essential salt solution dangled above their heads; doctors and nurses busily took blood pressures and vital signs while checking the cutdown sites to make sure that the saline and intravenous penicillin were gaining access to the body. Meanwhile, smiling flight attendants in their crisp red uniforms offered fruit juices and water to those patients able to drink from straws. Consul General Bennett and consulate medical officer Dr. Wolf were standing quietly off to the side, observing the work taking place aboard the plane.

To my surprise, Vic Thomas came aboard, accompanied by an elegantly dressed middle-aged Nigerian gentleman who was wearing a light brown gown and matching headgear—clothing often reserved for Sunday church attendance. Vic introduced him as Chief Jonathan Adis Obafemi Olopade, a chief in Lagos and one of several independent directors of Johnson–Nigeria. Chief Olopade (pronounced Oh-lop-a-day) was about fifty years old, an engineer, and the managing director of Adeladico Engineering in Lagos, a firm that primarily provided consulting services. Everyone's reaction as the chief strode down the aisle offering condolences and a blessing to each patient was like that of an awestruck Englishman bowing gracefully before his king or queen. The morale of the conscious patients soared.

While the chief visited the patients, Dr. Fairhurst assembled the medical team in the rear of the plane and complemented them on what they had already accomplished that morning, despite their lack of sleep over the last twenty-four hours. The somber-faced doctors nodded, and the nurses beamed. Next, Dr. Fairhurst outlined how he wished the team to function during the upcoming twelve- to thirteen-hour flight to the United States. The medical team would be divided into two groups, each group working a two-hour shift while the other group rested, ate, and slept. This approach, he believed, would provide the best possible patient care under the circumstances.

Of the sixteen patients presently on board, thirteen had systemic infections for which they had not been receiving adequate doses of antibiotics and were teetering on the threshold of death. Seven were in early kidney failure and suffering from hypovolemic shock. Only two, Allison

More Delays: Lagos—Saturday, Noon

Ehiemere and Hycenth Munonyi, were comfortably stable. However, until the debridement and skin grafting surgeries were completed, both remained in jeopardy of acquiring a serious systemic infection best prevented in the hygienic setting of a burn center.

Severe burns cause many complex systemic changes, the most significant of which in the early post-burn period is the alteration of fluid balance commonly referred to as fluid shift or burn shock. In a severe burn, the inflammation and fluid shift may be so marked as to cause hypovolemic shock that, if untreated, culminates in death. To avoid this deadly shock now present in the majority of our patients, we were doing our best to combat it with fluid therapy. Dr. Feller was concerned that many of the more severely burned Nigerians were critically dehydrated and as a result were on the brink of hypovolemic shock. This was why he had advised us to intravenously administer one liter of normal saline immediately to each of the Nigerians as soon as they were aboard the jet—this would hopefully keep them all alive until we reached Michigan. (Once the victims were in the Michigan burn center, the staff could quickly determine the degree of hypovolemia while they obtained blood cultures to specifically identify any invading bacteria. Then the infectious disease specialists would inform us as to the best antibiotic regime to initiate. These specialists would also be of immense help in identifying and treating any other common underlying diseases that could affect the outcome—such as diabetes, malaria, yellow fever, ascaris (roundworms), and schistosomiasis. In addition, the assistance of a nephrologist, with the hemodialysis artificial kidneys to combat the kidney failure in some of our patients, would be a godsend.)

The somber ambience in the passenger compartment was suddenly interrupted by a hideous scream of pain from John Akalamna, patient number 1, the factory worker who had regained consciousness after the rectally administered saline. He was in extreme pain and was begging for a Muslim cleric. A nurse quickly administered another dose of narcotic, and the young man slipped into a semisomnolent state. I suspected that the young factory worker's intuition of his impending death was correct, yet it hadn't occurred to me to inquire whether these patients had been visited by a Muslim, Protestant, or Catholic chaplain during their hospitalization.

At 1:45 PM, the tardy ambulance finally arrived, and the last two patients were hastily boarded. Patient number 17, Victor Akalona, was a twenty-five-year-old casual worker with 47 percent total body burns, most of which appeared to be partial thickness. However, his temperature was a high 104°F. Invading bacteria were threatening to prove fatal.

Patient number 18, Friday Omonuwas, was a thirty-two-year-old operator with 47 percent total body burns. Many of these were reported to be full thickness. As expected, he too had a high fever—another potential casualty during our upcoming flight. The disquieting image of a giant DC-10 landing at the Detroit airport and quietly unloading eighteen stretchers each bearing a heavily bandaged corpse flashed through my mind.

Following Dr. Feller's recommendation, these last patients were given IV fluids and penicillin once on board. By now, we were playing against the odds and racing against time.

By 2:20 PM, we were finally ready for departure. All visitors had deplaned, and the medical staff had taken their seats and fastened their seat belts. John Akalamna was semi-comatose and oblivious to the increasing roar of the jet engines as the DC-10 raced down the runway. I wondered what those who were aware of the noise were thinking. I glanced out the side window and noted the intensity of the rain beating down on the concrete. When we lifted off, I breathed a sigh of relief. *Finally!* And once the green jungle with its palm trees inserting themselves above the thick green underbrush dropped away from view, I silently whispered, "Good-bye, Africa." Overhead, the IV bottles hanging from clotheslines swayed from the motion of the jet. Each bottle had a needle in its vent; and as we ascended, the interior pressure in the jet would drop, and the bottles would begin to eject water like a lawn sprinkler.

Moments later I heard an ominous gasping sigh from Sibastian Onyensa, the young man with burns over half his body. I looked across the aisle at him. His body stiffened and gave several jerks, displacing the lightweight plastic oxygen mask over his nose and mouth. Ignoring the fasten seat belt sign, I slipped out of my seat and stepped to his side. He wasn't breathing, and I couldn't find a pulse. One of the doctors, joined by a nurse, rushed up to assist; we administered CPR—but to no avail. By the time the plane reached cruising altitude, I pronounced the young man dead and covered his blackened, swollen face with a white sheet. The looks of horror and fear on the faces of the conscious patients followed us as we carried the dead man on his stretcher down the aisle toward the front of the passenger compartment. Trying our best not to display any emotion, we secured the stretcher with the sheet-covered face on two of the vacant seats, now our designated morgue.

Ten minutes later, the doctor who had helped me administer CPR leaped out of his seat and dashed forward a couple of rows to join Dr. Fairhurst and a nurse administering CPR to Lambert Okpara. I remained in my seat clenching my teeth and silently repeating what I wished I could be shouting: *Hang in there! Don't give up! You can make it!* All to no avail. He too died, and I watched as a white sheet was pulled up over his face. This was worse than the most terrifying of nightmares—at least after a nightmare you can return to a sense of normalcy.

Dr. Fairhurst looked at his watch and dismissed two doctors and two nurses to the rear of the plane to eat and rest for two hours. He pointed to me and invited me to join them. I shook my head no. He nodded and replied in a low voice, that he would not hesitate to call me anytime he needed my assistance. I answered with an affirmative nod.

After dictating my notes into the tape recorder, I entered the first-class compartment to check on Jim Keane. He was seated, trying to read a newspaper and sipping a cup of Dutch-brewed coffee. He seemed relaxed, but he had been busy helping the others get the patients settled. After he saw the expression on my face, he gestured toward the passenger compartment and said he had the feeling that things weren't going too well back there.

I nodded and slumped into the seat across the aisle from Jim. "Two have died already," I replied. "I anticipated a number of deaths during the flight, but two in the first few minutes—it ties your gut in knots." Keane told me I looked beat and better catch forty winks while I could. I nodded and eased my seat into a semi-recumbent position. Before I closed my eyes, I dictated one more note, "Flight time to

More Delays: Lagos—Saturday, Noon

Detroit, nonstop, is estimated to be eleven and a half to twelve and a half hours, depending on the weather. This puts us there sometime around 8:00 to 9:00 PM Michigan time. Surprisingly, though, I've had but thirteen and one-half hours of interrupted sleep over the last four nights; I do feel alert and awake. It must be the adrenaline."

A flight attendant entered carrying a tray and offered me coffee in a delicate china cup reserved for first-class passengers. I sat up, adding sugar and cream. The first few sips of the delicious brew were lifesaving. Keane commented that the coffee was mighty tasty.

"Sure is, Jim." I set my cup down and leaned back in my seat. "Now to bed, to sleep—and not to dream."

CHAPTER 13

Over the Atlantic: Saturday Afternoon and Evening

Once we were airborne, I dozed for less than an hour until I was awakened by a vivid dream. In it I witnessed a trapeze artist falling from her swing in a crowded circus tent. She screamed shrilly as she plummeted. I instantly opened my eyes and lay there, listening intently for screaming from one of the burn patients in the passenger compartment behind me. I believed that some piercing noise must have triggered my dream. Two minutes passed. I heard nothing—all was quiet. The only noise reaching my ears was the muted, low-pitched hum of the jet engines.

I sat up and looked around the first-class compartment. In the seat across the aisle from me, Jim Keane was comfortably snoozing. Slowly I eased myself into the aisle and visited the restroom, speculating how Sigmund Freud would have interpreted my dream. I could picture the white-haired psychoanalyst slowly shaking his head and muttering that while I was doing as much as I could under the circumstances, this was not enough to stave off the impending disaster—a plane full of dead bodies. *Enough of the nightmare and negative thoughts!* I silently scolded myself. *Continue doing all that you can for the patients.*

I made my way to the passenger compartment and surveyed the scene. The medical team members were busily attending to the patients. Dr. Fairhurst looked up and signaled that all was under control. I nodded appreciatively and made my way to the seat occupied by Allison Ehiemere. He didn't appear to be in pain, and the IV I had started was still running smoothly.

While Allison was the least severely burned of our patients and the most likely to survive, his return to a near-normal life was going to be a long, tedious trek. To surgically reduce and, hopefully, erase the scarring of his badly burned face and hands would be a monumental challenge for the most skillful plastic surgeon. Dark-skinned people form huge amounts of scar tissue that remolds the face and hands. When I stopped beside him, Allison looked up from his heavily bandaged, badly swollen face and nodded. I smiled and reintroduced myself.

"Yes, I know who you are," he replied. "You are the head Johnson doctor." I nodded and told him that I knew very little about the details of the butane gas explosion and, worse yet, precious little about the personal lives of those who had been burned. As soon as he felt up to the task, I would greatly appreciate his briefing me on these topics. He nodded, telling me that he was up for the task now and would like to go on record with what he had observed—in case he didn't have the chance later on. With his permission, I recorded segments of his reply with my Dictaphone.

As Allison spoke, the miserably unhappy expression on his swollen, charred face remained unchanged as he talked of that fateful morning when Oli One rushed in to tell him what was happening outside. I had heard the account of the disaster several times, but I sensed it would help Allison to talk about it.

"I saw that the gas pipeline adjacent to the wall was lying mangled and broken beneath two feet of water," he said, "with hordes of butane gas bubbles rushing to the surface. I was scared that a spark or a lightning flash could ignite the escaping gas into a giant fireball. Many of our employees standing in the rising water were mesmerized by the water streaming through the breach in the crumbling retaining wall. I waved my hands and ordered everyone not directly involved in repairing the broken gas pipeline to immediately evacuate the area.

"I instructed Oli One to send one of his technicians to cut off power from the main switchboard. I wanted to avoid a possible catastrophe of the entire tank farm catching fire and exploding, which could lead to the massive destruction of the numerous plants in the Isolo Industrial Estate.

"No sooner had I spoken when suddenly everybody in the area was engulfed in huge flames, including myself. The thought of my family losing me flashed through my mind. As confused as the situation was, I am proud of everyone for remaining relatively calm and hurrying to help their burned colleagues."

As Allison continued to tell me about his harrowing trip to the hospital and the lack of funding available to hospitals in the country, it became apparent to me that speaking with such a swollen face was very uncomfortable for him. When he reached a pause, I thanked him for the conversation and told him to get some rest.

As I continued walking down the aisle, giving each patient a quick visual assessment, I made a resolution to learn more about Allison—the circumstances that brought him to Johnson–Nigeria and how he met Margaret. But for now, he needed to rest, and I needed to check on the other patients.

Suddenly one of the flight attendants cried out for me to please come and look at something. The shrillness of her cry made me spin around to see what was transpiring. The flight attendant was standing opposite Okon Bassey. She was covering her mouth with her right hand as if she were about to vomit. Horror gripped her face. She staggered back away from the patient's stretcher and pointed down at his heavily bandaged head. She told me there was a worm, a big, fat, ugly worm crawling out of his nose.

I quickly stepped over and looked down at the patient. Indeed, there was a worm slowly squirming out from his nose—a full two inches of its body was exposed, and the head was wriggling like it was searching for something. I had never before witnessed such a scene. Reaching down I gently grasped the creature one inch below its head and slowly extracted its wiggling body. As I held up the five- to six-inch creature, I glanced at the faces of the two nurses and the three attendants who were witnessing the procedure. The nurses were grimacing; the flight attendants were in a temporary state of shock. None of us had ever before witnessed such a startling phenomenon. I bagged the worm for the pathology lab and explained that while I had only seen pictures of intestinal parasites, this one was simply a hungry roundworm that was searching for food in the patient's empty gastrointestinal tract. My small audience stood there frozen in shock. I motioned for them to return to their duties and went to the lavatory to wash my hands.

Upon my return to the makeshift burn unit, I noted that Dele Jacobs, the accounts clerk with more than half his body burned, was carrying on a conversation with one of the flight attendants between sips of orange juice from a glass she was holding. When he indicated to the woman that he had had enough, I moved to the side of his stretcher and studied the visible portion of his face staring up at me through white bandages concealing all but his eyes, nose, and mouth. Dele, not reassured by my previous words of encouragement, asked me once again if he was dying.

"You are very badly burned, but in the Michigan center, they have the best of everything to heal your body. They have saved people with far worse burns than you have." Dele didn't look convinced. He closed his swollen eyelids and turned away. "Dele, if we didn't think we could save your life, you wouldn't be on this plane to the United States." The swollen eyelids opened, and he turned and looked up at me, once again asking if he were dying. "Without the special care available in the burn center to which we are flying, you would die. No doubt about it. You would die. Now you have a chance to live." Dele lay still showing no emotion. "Your marriage to the young woman to whom you wish to write is doomed without the special treatment being offered at the University of Michigan Trauma Burn Center."

But Dele asked me if he would have terrible scars if he survived. He asked if he would look like a leper.

"Dr. Feller, the American doctor who examined you in the hospital, is one of best in the world at erasing burn scars." However, Dele once again asked if he would look like a leper.

"No, you will not. But the treatment necessary to repair your burned body won't be easy. It will take weeks of treatment in the hospital to transplant some of your healthy, unburned skin to cover all the severely burned areas, but—and this is the important thing to keep telling yourself—while some of the treatments will be painful, and it won't be possible to erase all the burn scars completely, the scars that are left will be scarcely visible. You will be able to return to Nigeria looking like the good-looking young man your fiancée will be proud to marry." Dele said that no woman in all of Nigeria ever loves and marries a man with burn scars because they are so ugly.

"Nigeria doesn't have the doctors who can erase burn scars. That's why we are flying you to America. We have doctors in the United States, like Dr. Feller, who erase ugly burn scars every day." When Dele told me he did not have much money, I reassured him that he was not paying for the hospitalization.

"Johnson–Nigeria is paying for the hospitalization—not you." When he asked how soon the burn scars would be erased, I told him it will take awhile. "Once we grow new skin to cover the burn areas that have no skin left, we can erase most of the remaining burn scars." When he asked how long that would take and told him weeks, maybe months. There was silence while he took this in.

Lacking the skills of a minister of God, I said, "Pray to your god to be with you and to help with your recovery." He told me he believed in Christ and that he would pray. In a quivering voice he told me he was born and grew up in Ghana, where his wife-to-be lives. He said sadly that he could not write to her with bandaged hands.

"We will help you. Now don't worry. Relax, rest, it will help you heal." Dele nodded and closed his eyes.

The thought struck me again as I walked away that in the absence of a proper cleric in our makeshift ICU, maybe I should be pausing to say a prayer at the stretcher of each of the burn victims. *No, I told myself. Every move a doctor makes to aid a patient is a prayer—a silent prayer—a doctor's prayer to the Creator of Life.*

At the bedside of Oli One—who had burns on his face, hands, torso, and thighs—I studied the especially severe burns on his left eyelid, ear, and his entire left forehead. To restore his facial features would be a titanic challenge left to the nimble fingers of Dr. Feller. Like Allison, Oli's English was superb, and he was eager to have someone with whom to talk. I learned that he was married and had four children—daughters ten and six and eight-year-old twins. He had studied chemistry for four years at the University of Ibadan, following which he had worked four years each for two large corporations before joining Johnson–Nigeria.

When the flooding began, Oli found himself standing in two and a half feet of rising water. By the time he and Allison had reached the crumbling retaining wall, the whole complex was engulfed in two gigantic fireballs. Oli was stunned to see 80 percent of his shirt completely burned off, exposing unnaturally colored skin with shreds of blackened cloth fragments embedded in it. Sixty percent of his trousers were also burned away. He stood there, dazed and naked in knee-deep water.

Standing next to him, the finance manager resembled a kerosene torch. Yellowish orange flames were devouring the heavy polyester business suit he had worn to impress Jim Keane at the morning meeting. The screaming manager had stumbled forward and collapsed in the water. He remembered Allison, rising up from his dive into the water and shouting at the top of his voice, "Please take the people to Ajanaku Hospital!" because he knew that the medical care provided there would be immediate.

He and five others, including Allison, were helped into a car for what should have been a thirty-minute drive to the hospital—but the incoming traffic was moving at a snail's pace. Like Allison had earlier, he told me of the frantic drive to the hospital. They had stopped briefly at a medical clinic in Isolo for emergency pain medication before continuing on for another hour to reach Ajanaku Hospital.

Oli One told me that it was during the drive that he became aware of the pain for the first time. It began with a creepy sensation arising in the burn areas that erased the initial numb sensation. This sensation gave way to real pain that steadily increased in intensity. By the time they reached the little hospital, the pain had become excruciatingly unbearable. He grimaced as he recalled the gruesome moments of severe pain, and then commented that while the pain was still troublesome, the medicine he was now receiving made it much more bearable.

I reassured Oli that he would be well cared for once he reached Michigan. As I left to visit another patient, I prayed that he would be fortunate enough to one day return home to the loving arms of his wife and children.

For me the long flight from Lagos to Detroit was an exhausting experience. My adrenaline-fueled energy had kept me going for the past few days in order to get the burn patients on their way to help. I hadn't had enough sleep, and now fatigue suddenly hit me, enhancing my concern about the potential survival rate of the patients on board. Of the twenty-four severely burned Nigerians, six had already died in the four days before the jumbo jet now serving as our emergency burn ICU arrived in Lagos. Of the remaining eighteen patients, two had died shortly after takeoff, four were teetering on death's doorstep, and five others were only a half-step behind.

Three hours into the flight, no one else had died, thankfully. We had slowed that avalanche at least. All the patients had received at least one liter of intravenous normal saline and two million units of penicillin. Dr. Fairhurst's two medical teams were performing exceptionally well. Team 2, with two doctors and two nurses, was now busy caring for patients, while team 1 was enjoying its first two-hour rest period.

All the flight attendants had overcome their abhorrence of the sight and smell of the burn patients and had joined in their care. With an encouraging smile, they gave oral fluids to the conscious patients, carefully recording on each chart the milliliters of fluid given. They also gave urine collection bottles to those able to urinate and recorded the urinary output. This was a completely spontaneous gesture on the part of the flight attendants because they wanted to help and not because they had been requested to do so by the doctors and nurses. We were all impressed by their kindness, professionalism, and willingness to pitch in and help in any way needed.

As the day wore on, sleep deprivation continued to take its toll on me despite the frequent cups of strong black coffee served by one of the ever-smiling attendants. On the several occasions when I found myself falling asleep on my feet, I made my way to the restroom in the first-class passenger compartment and splashed cold water on my face. Twice I simply had to slip into a seat, fasten the seat belt, lower the window blind, and shut my eyes. Sleep instantly swept over me, easing the tension and fatigue. Both times I was awakened within thirty to forty-five minutes—once by a jolt of air turbulence and a second time by an announcement from the cockpit requesting everyone to fasten their seat belts. The pilot said there was a fierce storm in our flight path and, in order to avoid a very bumpy ride and much discomfort to our patients, he would have to fly around it. This would add at least another hour or two to our already tediously long flight. Feeling surprisingly rejuvenated after my short second nap, I returned to our intensive care compartment, pausing to carefully study each patient's medical chart. Dr. Fairhurst's two medical teams were continuing to perform exceptionally well.

Keeping a perpetual smile on my face, I stopped to chat and bolster the morale of those patients who were conscious. This was particularly difficult with the four patients who were teetering on death's doorstep. The youngest, twenty-year-old Paul Oquamanam, had a soaring fever and was in septic shock. K. K. Olamayin was also in septic shock.

It appeared that his entire head had full-thickness burns. I had never read about survival in such a case—the months of skin transplantation and plastic surgeries required would be monumental. The third critically ill patient, Badu Dada, not only had a high fever indicative of a horrible widespread infection but also had an abnormally slow pulse rate and pulmonary edema (fluid in the lungs blocking oxygen transport). The fourth of the critically ill was Oyebanji Adekola, the twenty-three-year-old quality-control manager with 46 percent of his body burned. He had extensive pneumonia in both lungs and was in kidney failure. I doubted he would still be alive when we arrived at the burn center. We needed immediate access to an artificial kidney to keep him alive, plus a clinical laboratory to identify the best antibiotics to administer to eradicate the bacteria causing his pneumonia.

When we were only two hours from the Detroit Metropolitan Airport, I obtained a direct voice link with Irv at the burn center. I briefed him on the present status of the patients, and he in turn informed me that all was in readiness. Two Jolly Green Giants, staffed by members of the 501st U.S. Air Force Search and Rescue Squadron, were awaiting our arrival at Detroit and would transport the patients to the burn center. Each helicopter was capable of carrying twelve stretchers. Doctors and nurses from the burn care staff were also there to join the military in the triage of the patients as they were transferred to a helicopter and to continue patient care during the short flight to the burn center.

I returned to my seat after briefing Dr. Fairhurst on my conversation with Irv. For me, this tedious day would finally end when the plane landed in Detroit and all the patients were handed over to Irv and his burn team. His task of wrenching as many as possible from the clutch of death would be monumental!

But a sudden bump reminded me again of the detour we were taking around the electrical storm—a storm that could prove deadly if we were to get any closer to it. I felt a shudder of fear run through my spine and silently hoped that we had enough fuel to stay in the air for the additional hours needed to avoid the catastrophic storm. I leaned back in my seat, my seat buckle clicking slightly during each turbulent jerk of the aircraft, and felt my stomach rise and fall during each air pocket. *We have to make it through this weather*, I thought. *This is the last chance for saving these poor people.*

CHAPTER 14

Touchdown in Detroit, Michigan: Saturday, 9:15 PM

To avoid any delay in our arrival, all incoming and outgoing flights from the Detroit Metropolitan Airport had been suspended until our DC-10 landed. Our pilot made a magnificently smooth landing without any braking or reverse thrust. I noted that there was a fire engine and an ambulance on each runway turnoff, instructed to follow the aircraft down the runway to the stand where the helicopters were waiting. Later I was told that the plane's fuel supply was precariously low and that this was the reason for all the precautions.

As soon as the airplane came to a full stop, two medical teams on two high lifts rushed into the plane to begin unloading patients. I glanced out of the window and noted that a small group of spectators had moved up to within thirty yards of the aircraft. In front of the crowd were Bob Petersen and my boss, Bill Eastham. Soon I would be able to walk up to them and shake their hands, thanking them for helping to successfully pull off an almost-impossible mission. We now had a good chance to save a significant number of lives that otherwise would have been lost.

Loading the patients off the plane was completed in less than an hour, except for the bodies of the two men who died during the flight. Once all the patients were off the aircraft, the flight attendants, who had been under tremendous stress, began to finally relax; some even bantered with members of the 501st Air Force Search and Rescue Squadron. (Later I learned that road ambulances arrived later that evening and off-lifted the two bodies from the plane. An hour later, the refueled DC-10 departed Detroit with two new and rested pilots for the return flight to Holland, arriving twenty-five hours and thirty minutes after its initial departure.)

I breathed a sigh of relief when the two helicopters carrying the surviving sixteen Nigerians lifted up from the airport into the darkening evening sky and headed for the burn center in Ann Arbor. Soon these badly burned survivors would be in the hands of some of the most skillful burn care doctors and nurses in the country. Hopefully, their life-threatening infections would be quelled, allowing the large areas of damaged skin to be initially replaced with healthy donor skin, permitting them to resume a healthy recovery, free from bacterial invasion.

I was then informed that a driver was available to rush me to the burn center once I had passed through customs and immigration. When I exited the passenger terminal, an attendant met me and insisted on carrying my luggage while he led me to the waiting car. The driver stepped out of the Buick LeSabre and opened the rear door for me. I eased myself back into one of the luxurious seats, and for the first time in five long days and nights, I was able to fully relax. I had done what I could do for the victims. Now it was up to the burn center to save their lives. Leaning back, I closed my eyes. Sleep soon overcame me, and I dozed soundly until the driver stopped at the entrance to the burn center and opened the door for me to exit.

I had never been inside the new University of Michigan Trauma Burn Center or witnessed their care for seriously burned patients in the nation, though I had heard colleagues discuss the center's merits and its sterling accomplishments. The center was renowned for having saved the lives of the very young and the elderly with 80 to 90 percent total body burns. Thinking about this restored my optimism for our Nigerian patients—they were healthy young adults, and even though we were three to four days late in arrival, the center still had a fighting chance to work its lifesaving magic.

Before I was allowed to enter the brightly illuminated and completely sterile triage and emergency care section of the center, I was directed to the physicians' quarters, given a locker in which to store my clothing, and shown where I could shower before slipping into clean surgical garments. All these precautions were to prevent the myriad of bacteria on me and my clothing from coming into contact with the patients in the ward.

For me the scene in the triage and emergency care section was something out of a science fiction film. Each of the near-to-death patients was lying on a brightly illuminated surgical bed. At the bedside of each, two surgeons and two nurses similarly garbed in operating room attire were busily engaged in the initial emergency care. Lifesaving intravenous fluid was streaming down through plastic tubes from overhead IV bags dangling from thin steel poles firmly attached to the surgical beds. Blood and urine specimens were being collected and handed to technicians, who immediately hurried the samples to the various laboratories for prompt processing. Identifying the specific life-threatening bacteria invading and feeding on the victims would allow the staff to administer the appropriate antibiotics.

Overseeing each patient's care and making lightning-fast decisions was the burn center's commanding officer—Irv Feller. I stood off to the side, slipped my Nikon camera out of its case, and prepared to photograph this spectacular scene.

Suddenly there was a scurry of activity around the surgical table where Badu Dada, the twenty-one-year-old with over 60 percent total body burns—from his head to his thighs—lay. He had a temperature of 104°F, a sky-high blood pressure, and was severely dehydrated. He was intubated and a CVP line inserted for vigorous fluid rehydration. Then his blood pressure began to fall, and his pulse rate progressively slowed. Suddenly he went into cardiac arrest.

I edged closer and watched the tall doctor towering over the patient place two defibrillator paddles on the man's chest and deliver an electrical shock. The young man's body stiffened for a fraction of a second then relaxed. His heart didn't respond, and there was no pulse. The doctor signaled to his colleagues to stand back, then delivered a second stronger electrical shock into his limp body. Again the body stiffened for a fraction of a second, and this time his heart awakened and resumed beating slowly. The doctor relayed the information, that the pulse rate was forty per minute. Blood pressure was sixty over forty.

Touchdown in Detroit, Michigan: Saturday, 9:15 PM

One of the assisting nurses, noting my presence, turned her head and said softly that septicemia with a temperature of 104°F indicated severe pulmonary edema from heart failure.

After the severe burn had destroyed half of his protective full-thickness skin, bacteria had invaded his body. Over the past four days, the bacteria had multiplied. Now millions of microscopic germs were having a field day feasting on all parts of his body. The massive dose of antibiotics he was now receiving was slaughtering the bacteria in record numbers, but not in time to undo the widespread injury that had already occurred in many of his internal organs. His bacteria-ravaged heart was beating poorly, allowing fluid to flood into the myriad of tiny air sacs in his lungs, reducing the essential oxygen supply he so desperately needed. I feared I was viewing a man who might be taking his last breaths.

According to my list of patients, given to me as I boarded the plane in Nigeria, this young man's next of kin was his brother. He was not married. *At least he would not be leaving a wife and children behind to mourn*, I determined, though it didn't make his situation any less hard to swallow.

There were hushed voices at the adjacent surgical table where K. K. Olamayin lay. I stepped closer to view the brisk activity. The man had sustained 64 percent burns, and he too was in septic shock. Heroic measures were being taken to pull him back to life, but death appeared to be winning. I recalled that this man did have a wife listed as his next of kin, and I wondered if he had children that would soon be left without a father.

Nearby, Oyebanji Adekola, the quality-control manager, with 46 percent total burns from head to legs, also appeared to be slipping away. Bacteria had strolled into the parts of his body lacking protective skin and had taken up housekeeping in both of his lungs. The concentration of the available oxygen in the circulating blood had dropped into the danger zone. Now his heart was weakening, and the tiny blood vessels throughout his body were beginning to clot, further disrupting blood flow. His kidneys had also ceased functioning. The outlook was dire.

I continued making my rounds, marveling at the immense care being administered to each individual man. Even though everything possible was being done, there were about seven or eight Nigerians whom I feared might expire in the next twenty-four hours. As I viewed the scene unfolding in the unit, I felt as though I was walking through a nightmare, witnessing the pitiful demise of a room full of young Nigerian men, all of whom could have survived had the proper medical care been immediately available.

I felt a sense of agony viewing those who were dying around me, but I was also in awe of the marvelous efforts that were under way to save as many as could be saved. It was at that moment that I firmly resolved to review the current disaster preparedness programs in place for each of the fifty-four SC Johnson facilities around the world, in case such a tragedy struck once again. While I wasn't responsible for any of these operations, I felt honor-bound to investigate and make recommendations where local standards didn't meet those in place for U.S. employees. In Racine, we held periodic personnel drills simulating what best to do in the event of a tornado, a fire, a flood, or a gas explosion like the one in Nigeria. If the subsidiaries didn't already have measures like this in practice, I wanted to help make sure they would in the near future.

Touchdown in Detroit, Michigan: Saturday, 9:15 PM

As I looked over the emergency triage area, I counted only fourteen surgical teams at work. Two patients were missing: Allison Ehiemere and Okon Bassey. I nervously approached one of the senior nurses and inquired what had happened to these two. To my relief, I was told that Dr. Feller requested both men transported to the Chelsea Community Hospital burn facility, one of the perimeter backup burn care units whose staff was personally trained by Irv. The nurse commented thatCed Dr. Feller felt these two patients had a good chance for total recovery; thus, they didn't require the intensive burn therapy the other fourteen patients in the burn center were now receiving.

Even though these two were supposedly "out of the woods," Allison would require a talented plastic surgeon to successfully mend his body (primarily his face and hands) so he could return to normal life in Nigeria. Okon Bassey's burns on his head and torso were, thankfully, only partial thickness, which meant they did not require extensive skin grafting. The primary focus of his care, then, was to stave off additional infections.

I glanced at the clock hanging on the wall. It was far too late to travel the fifteen to twenty miles to the Chelsea Community Hospital to check on Allison and Okon, so I resolved to do so the first thing in the morning.

At 11:00 PM, I left the bustling activity in the burn care center and made my way to my hotel room. Just maybe, I thought, this center would be able to pluck a few of the fourteen Nigerians from death.

The dictated note I muttered that night before bed stated, "Midnight. I drop into bed totally exhausted. This has been an unbelievable day!"

CHAPTER 15

Ann Arbor, Michigan: Sunday Morning

As I showered early Sunday morning, I looked up at the hot water streaming down from the showerhead, closed my eyes, and stepped into the warm downpour. The water massaged and refreshed my body. Standing quietly there in the warmth of the running water, I planned my day. First, I would contact Irv and get an update on all the Nigerian patients, beginning with the two I had yet to visit in the Chelsea Community Hospital. Then I would relay both the good and the bad news to the key SC Johnson managers and directors in both Racine and Nigeria. I suspected that Bob Peterson was eager to establish a daily medical report communication system with Dr. Feller, so today I would do what I could to expedite the process. I too wanted to stay informed once I returned to Racine in a few days.

I managed to reach Irv by phone before he began his morning rounds. He sounded wide awake although

I suspected he had had only a few hours of restful sleep. He updated me on all the Nigerians beginning with the one fatality they'd had overnight. I immediately suspected it was Badu Dada, the twenty-one-year-old, whose cardiac arrest I had witnessed the night before. I was right. The young man had experienced a second cardiac arrest shortly before midnight, this time nonreversible, losing the battle to overcome the overwhelming septicemia that had seized him. Regrettably, our efforts to save his life had been too late.

Irv said that as of this morning, the survival of five of the Nigerian patients was still questionable. Despite the efforts of the burn center staff to utilize every available medical measure to pull these five away from death, kidney failure and high fevers from overwhelming bacterial infections were proving to be almost fatal. Eight other patients, while still critical, had better than a fifty-fifty chance of survival. The bright exceptions were the two patients in the Chelsea Community Hospital burn facility. Allison Ehiemere would probably be ready for split-thickness skin grafts for his hands and ears within a week to ten days. Okon Bassey, with only partial-thickness burns, would luckily heal and require only minimal skin grafting.

Irv paused, broke the mounting tension with a chuckle, and told me that Allison's "amazing wife" had managed to get onto a flight from Nigeria and was now at her husband's bedside. Since her arrival at the Chelsea Community Hospital, Margaret had become a valuable member of Irv's burn team, he confided in me. One of the first things she had done to raise the morale of her husband and Okon was to inform the dietitians how to prepare their meals in a Nigerian style. For the first time since the fiery explosion, the two men had smiles on their faces when breakfast was served. Margaret fascinated me, and I was set on talking with her later that day.

When I arrived at the Chelsea Community Hospital later that morning, I found that both Allison and Okon had undergone rigorous burn-wound cleansing upon their arrival, had experienced a restful night of sleep, and were now lying in bed clothed in bulky dressings. The two were fully bandaged and wide awake; and after having had a good Nigerian-style breakfast, they were bracing themselves for another day of burn-wound care, but this time with smiles on their faces.

Margaret Ehiemere, a woman with sparkling, expressive eyes, was seated in a chair next to her husband's bed. She stood up and welcomed me with a cheerful "Good morning, Dr. Stewart" and, uninhibited, gave me a hug. "Thank you so much for getting Allison and the others to where they are now receiving good treatment for their burns. You have saved their lives!"

"No, Margaret," I replied, "it was Allison's quick response to the explosion and his getting the burn victims to hospitals—plus Jim Keane's call for help—that saved their lives. Had Allison and Jim not done what they did, there would have been far too many premature funerals."

This introductory conversation opened the door for me to learn more about Margaret and Allison. Over the weeks and months that followed, my admiration for them and what they were doing in their community soared.

Allison Ehiemere was born and raised in Eziala-Nsulu, Isiala Ngwa, in Eastern Nigeria. His father was not considered incredibly wealthy, but the family was, nonetheless, upper middle class and his father became a well-respected member of the Eziala-Nsulu community. This afforded Allison the funds with which to attend the Methodist College at Uzuakoli, Eastern Nigeria, at a time when fewer than 5 percent of the elementary school population attended college. After graduation in 1960, he had worked for a brief period in the Produce Inspection Division of the Eastern Nigeria Ministry of Agriculture and then for three years as a sales representative at the Nigerian Tobacco Company, rising to the position of sales supervisor.

Allison confessed to me that as a young man, he had aspirations to achieve far more in life than his position as a sales supervisor for a tobacco company. His ultimate goal was to rise to a position in life that would enable him to help his people cast off the shackles of ignorance and poverty and realize their full potential. However, to achieve this mission, he realized that he first needed a higher-quality education, so he applied for admission to a number of colleges in the United States.

Westmar College in Le Mars, Iowa, was the first to offer him admission and a four-year scholarship. He was an excellent student, and all went well. During the school year, he worked part-time in Westmar for pocket money; and during his four summer vacations, he worked full-time, first in Texas, then in Connecticut, and finally in Michigan—"to learn as much as possible about the USA."

While working in Detroit, Allison met his wife, Margaret, who was studying at Wayne State University. She had grown up in Camden, South Carolina, and came to Detroit where her older sister—a school librarian—lived. Margaret graduated from Felician Academy, a Catholic girls' school, attended Madonna College, and transferred to Wayne State

University from which she graduated in December 1970. She was immediately employed as a science teacher.

Allison graduated from Westmar College in June 1970, and he married Margaret two months later. During their courtship, though, he had confided in Margaret about the atrocities happening in his home country—the ongoing three-year civil war that had devastated his family in Igboland—and so the pair decided to forego a "traditional" wedding and sent as much financial assistance as they could to facilitate his family's rehabilitation in Nigeria.

Allison's first job after graduation was as a sales representative for J. Lewis Cooper Company, a wine distributor in Detroit. Two years later, he joined SC Johnson as a sales representative. Here he took advantage of the company's educational assistance program and graduated from the University of Detroit with an MBA in May 1976. Margaret earned her master's degree in education from Wayne State the following December.

Offered a sales and marketing manager position at the SC Johnson subsidiary in Nigeria, Allison was delighted by the opportunity to return to the country and family he loved. In January 1977, after six months of training in the SC Johnson regional office in Surrey, England, Allison and family arrived in Lagos, Nigeria. Vic Thomas, the general manager of Johnson–Nigeria at the time, did much to facilitate a smooth transition for this young family into a totally new social environment. He made it possible for Allison's three children to attend Corona School, Gbagada, the former British elementary school for American children.

Eighteen months after Allison's arrival in Nigeria, Vic was promoted to area director and transferred to the regional office in England. Allison, the second in command in 1978, stepped up into Vic's position as general manager. Under Allison's guidance, I later learned, the company expanded and developed and went from locally manufacturing 25 percent of its annual sale's products to locally manufacturing 80 percent. This saved the company from suffering too gravely during Nigeria's period of economic downturn in the '70s and '80s, which was due to the scarcity of hard currency and the restriction of importing finished products for resale. Consequently, Nigeria–Johnson was enjoying "good health" compared to most other companies in the country at the time.

"We were looking forward to an even better future," Allison commented, "when suddenly everything changed overnight—on that fateful day."

Margaret told me it had been nothing less than a blessed morning. A damp Monday in the rainy season—it seemed that it had rained all weekend. She had been alone with the children for most of the time. Allison had attended the funeral of Mr. Isangadighi, the company's marketing manager, in the eastern part of the country. Upon his return from the funeral, Allison and Margaret had discussed the tragedy of Mr. Isangadighi's death and the beautiful family he left behind. That Monday, as Allison left for work, Margaret said that she held her husband close before saying good-bye. She felt a sense of gratefulness and joy in her life at that moment.

"I will always remember my trip to the open market that morning," Margaret shared with me. "Shopping in the open market in many developing countries can be a social event. In Nigeria I had my sellers from whom I usually purchased things. We haggled prices every week as we postured, teased, intimidated, and agreed on what I would pay. As I jumped over puddles to enter other stalls, I was amused by my deep sense of well-being in the market, in the country, and in my world.

"I prayed a prayer of gratitude for the way things were working out for me and my family in Nigeria. The children were doing well in school. Chisara was at Queen's College, generally considered the premier girls' institution in the country. Abazie was taking first place in reading at Corona School Gbagaga, an excellent elementary school by any world standard. Enyi was just a happy child, climbing the security gates and visiting the boys' quarter, without my knowledge, to have morning tea with our driver and his uncles who lived behind our house."

Margaret said she was completing a year on leave from the University of Lagos at the University of Ibadan, located at the International Center for Educational Evaluation, hopeful that she would be able to continue to contribute to the educational advancement of Nigeria's civilians. She experienced success publishing the revised edition of the Science Teachers Association of Nigeria's *Integrated Science*.

After Margaret had finished her shopping and was just arriving home (to the house they had lived in for the past four years), she noticed her husband's driver, John, standing at the gate next to his yellow, duck-colored Peugeot. "He reminded me of a pet dog who had lost his master, with his body bent over and shaking." John moved deliberately and slowly opened the gate so that Margaret could park inside. "John looked at me with sad eyes, seeming unable to speak. I had always feared the tank farm at Johnson Wax. I knew that workers at the plant faced the danger of the butane catching fire. Quietly, which is not my style, I asked a simple question, 'Is it the tank farm?'"

"'No, madam.'

"'Has there been a fire?'

"'Yes, madam.'

"'Is he alive?'

"'Yes, madam.'

"'Let's go. You can tell me more on the way.'"

During the five-minute drive to Ajanaku Hospital, John tried to prepare Margaret for what she was about to witness, but upon seeing her husband's face covered in what she described as a blackened "mask," it was too much for her: "I started to scream a scream that I was unable to get out. Just as I started, Allison hushed me in a way that only he could have done. 'This is not the time for crying,' he told me. 'There is much to be done.'"

Thus began a chaotic week for Margaret. "Things to do and not to do, demons to pray away and poisons to avoid, fluids that Allison could drink while others dehydrated and died, missed opportunities to send for a priest, food delivered by friends, friends protecting my children, friends finding airline tickets, and in only the greatest Nigerian humor, a friend reassuring Allison that all was not lost because his sexual organ was not burned!"

Margaret slept at the hospital on a mattress that was brought from home. Most of all, because of her fear of Allison becoming dehydrated, she forced him to drink liquids; in fact, she forced him to imbibe so much Ribena—a liquid form of nutrients, produced by a pharmaceutical company, with a less-than-desirable flavor—that he vowed he'd never drink the liquid again in his life.

Ann Arbor, Michigan: Sunday Morning

When Margaret learned that a plane was coming to take the victims to the burn care center at the University of Michigan, she contacted her sister Jimmie in Detroit so she would have a place to stay as well as the transportation to get to Ann Arbor. Her sons, ages two and eight, came with her, but she had to leave her high school–aged daughter in Nigeria to finish out the semester.

"Jimmie and her husband met the boys and me at the airport on that June 26 Sunday evening. It was already dark, so the time would have been after 10:00 PM. We drove straight to the University of Michigan Trauma Burn Center. A nurse, looking at the list of new patients, could not find Allison's name. 'Some died on the flight,' she concluded. 'He must have been one of them.'

"I saw my sister almost pass out, but I did not blink. It was as if I was outside of the situation looking back at us. I was annoyed that the nurse could have been so callous, but I was determined to find my husband. I had seen the patients after they had been boarded in Lagos, and Allison was one of the strongest, so the thought of foul play crossed my mind. Most of Allison's family and friends had been concerned with him being poisoned at the hospital, but I quickly threw that thought away. Eventually I learned that some of the patients who were less seriously burned had been taken to Chelsea. So back on the road in the midnight darkness we drove the twenty miles to the Chelsea Community Hospital, where we found Allison and Okon Bassey wrapped in bandages and in pain, but hopeful of surviving."

CHAPTER 16

Hoping for Miracles:
Ann Arbor—Sunday Afternoon

After the morning session at the Chelsea Community Hospital, I briefly stopped at the University of Michigan Medical Library and approached one of the librarians seated behind the checkout desk. The white-haired woman behind the desk looked up and greeted me with a broad smile. I explained that I was a colleague of Dr. Feller's and asked if I could see any journals or information about the current treatment of severe burns.

The librarian told me that I was in luck, and led me to what she called the best book currently available. I followed her to one shelf loaded with volumes of textbooks. She stopped in the section labeled surgery and pulled a thick brown leather-bound volume from a shoulder-high shelf and handed it to me. She said it was published in 1979 by the National Institute for Burn Medicine two and a half years ago—*Reconstruction and Rehabilitation of the Burned*

Patient—and one of the editors and authors is none other than your Dr. Feller. She pointed to one of the empty reading tables and told me to have a seat and check it over and also mentioned that it was available in their bookstore.

I scanned the heavy book—423 thick pages filled with multiple photographs, charts, and drawings, 119 chapters written by sixty-nine physicians and burn care specialists from the most prestigious medical facilities in the world. As I browsed the book, I was surprised to see Irv's name listed next to the title of president of the National Institute for Burn Medicine. This was news to me.

I returned *Reconstruction and Rehabilitation of the Burned Patient* to the librarian, thanked her, and headed for the bookstore to purchase my own copy. I wanted to learn all I could in order to be as much help as possible to the patients and, also, be able to inform the executives at SC Johnson about all that was required in caring for these patients.

As I entered the burn center later that morning to check on the most severely burned of our Nigerian patients, I took a deep breath and braced myself for any bad news about the overnight survival of the patients. Gowned in a spotless surgical top, trousers, and shoe covers, I stepped inside the intensive care unit. The quiet hustle and bustle of the doctors and nurses caring for the patients was even more intense than I had observed the evening before.

The head nurse, dressed in white surgical garb and wearing a surgical face mask, spotted me and came to my side. She lowered her mask to better brief me on the status of the patients. The bad news was that several more Nigerians would probably die despite the extraordinary efforts of the medical staff to save them. Before repositioning her face mask, she handed me a mask as well, in order to protect the patients from any additional, and possible life-threatening, bacteria.

The nurse commented what a shame it was that these patients were not given the proper treatment during the emergent period—the first twenty-four to forty-eight hours after the accident—of their burns. As I well knew, the emergent period is considered the most critical period for beginning lifesaving burn therapy. During these first two days, the objective in all burn patients is to resolve the problems of fluid imbalance and to stabilize the body systems of the patient through debridement, fluid therapy, and dressing changes. Unfortunately for the Nigerian burn victims, these first critical days had been lost due to the lack of resources in the Nigerian hospitals and the increased time it took for us to bring them to Michigan.

When full-thickness skin burns occur, that portion of the burned skin becomes a leathery mass of dead tissue into which essential fluids from the body escape. This dead tissue is called *eschar*. Worst of all, the burned skin has lost all ability to fend off the bacteria that normally live on the surface of the skin. Without the proper defense, the skin is exposed to all germs it comes into contact with, and these bacteria can now enter and feast on the organs and tissues of the body.

Debridement, the removal of eschar, is necessary to prepare a clean surface of granulation tissue that will accept skin grafts, sealing the wound from bacterial invasion. The sooner this is accomplished, the less chance there will be for septicemia to develop due to any bacteria invading the body.

Debridement is initially carried out following admission to a burn care facility and is then performed daily at the time of dressing changes.

The size and depth of a patient's skin burns are key factors in determining the magnitude of the many complex systemic changes taking place throughout the body. The most significant of these in the early post burn period is the alteration of fluid balance, commonly referred to as *fluid shift* or *burn shock*. In a severe full-thickness burn, the patient's wound may be very large and the resulting fluid shift so marked as to cause *hypovolemic shock*, which, if not treated properly, will lead to death, as it did for a few of the Nigerians.

Dressings also serve many important purposes: they prevent contact transmission of bacteria, they speed up wound debridement, they protect granulation tissue and new grafts from bacteria, and they help conserve body heat and fluids.

As we entered the ward, the nurse pointed toward one of the desperately ill Nigerians and led the way with short hurried steps to his bedside over which dangled several IV bottles. Huddled around the bed was a team of three doctors and two nurses engaged in external cardiac massage to restart his failing heart.

Reflexively, I gritted my teeth for a moment and then relaxed. *Just maybe he'll make it*, I thought. *It's a small chance, but just maybe.*

The nurse glanced at the wall clock and then, in a soft voice, told me that they had been at this for over forty minutes—intravenous fluid replacement, bicarbonate, epinephrine, and the current external cardiac massage—the works. She paused a moment and added that so far his spontaneous cardiac rhythm hadn't returned and she was afraid they were losing him.

All this was a gruesome sight. The bulky bandages holding his dressings in place so obscured his face and upper body that it was impossible for me to recognize him. The only part of his body visible was his uncovered chest, which had become a sheet of leathery eschar.

Later I found it was patient 13, Emmanuel Adeeko, who, at forty-seven, was one of the older factory workers and had over 50 percent of his head, torso, arms, thighs, buttocks, and left leg burned.

The nurse informed me that when the man arrived yesterday, he had a temperature of 105°F and was severely dehydrated. He was intubated and a CVP line inserted for vigorous fluid rehydration. His blood pressure became progressively lower, falling from 110 systolic to 60 when vasopressors were begun. Shortly after this time, he became anuric [kidney failure] and went on to cardiopulmonary arrest. The burn team was doing everything it could, but they were not sure it was enough.

The nurse gestured for us to proceed to the next of the severely ill patients. I stepped closer to her and whispered, "Dr. Feller did his best to instruct the Nigerian doctors on how to clean and dress the victims' severely burned skin the day before we put them on the plane for transport to the United States. We both knew that this was a belated attempt, but it did afford us a chance to save some of them."

While we were completing our rounds on the remaining thirteen seriously burned patients, we observed from a distance that the resuscitation efforts on Oyebanji Adekola had ended, his heart had failed to resume beating, a sheet had been pulled over his heavily bandaged head, and his body was being lifted onto a stretcher for removal to the morgue.

Another death! Another death! echoed within my brain.

I spent the remainder of the day observing the burn team's valiant effort to save lives. As I did so, I consoled myself with the thought that at least the two Nigerians at the Chelsea Community Hospital had a good chance for survival. Amazingly, eight of the eleven Nigerians whom I was fearful would die this Sunday had began to stabilize, and a small sunbeam of hope peeked through the dark clouds of my concern. The intensive antibiotic and fluid therapy were life jackets that were keeping their bobbing heads above water.

By midnight on that Sunday, only three of the Nigerians in critical condition had died. However, three days later, on June 30, patient number 12, Samuel Oluwasuyi, the casual worker with 65 percent total body burns, succumbed to the widespread bacterial invasion that had invaded his body. He had developed severe pneumonia and unstoppable gastrointestinal tract bleeding that led to heart failure and shock. Now there were only eight patients left, but thankfully, they were stable and improving daily.

While I was visiting the patients at the burn center's ICU, I noticed that Margaret had stepped into the role of our Nigerian patients' mother. After Allison's first meal at the Chelsea Community Hospital, he complained to Margaret that the food being served to him and the other patient was terrible and asked her to instruct the hospital dietitians as to what Nigerians should be served. Burn patients needed to consume a huge number of calories each day, and when queried by the dietitians what they would most like to eat, Allison Ehiemere and Okon Bassey had requested "rice, only rice." To their dismay, they had been served only plain rice; this was an example of a harmless cultural misunderstanding, as by "only rice," these patients had meant rice with a rich tomato sauce and including fish or meat—a staple Nigerian dish. Allison was even more concerned that the more severely burned patients at the burn care center were probably facing the same food dilemmas, and he asked Margaret to inform the dietitians at both institutions about Nigerian food preferences.

Margaret later told me, "I'm here for Allison, but he has encouraged me to visit with all the burn victims and build a cultural network for them. He is fearful that none of them will be able to tolerate the American diet that the hospitals are serving. The men know me as Oga's wife, the Oyibo *dudu*, the black white woman, recognizing my American birth, and I have promised to do as he wishes."

Margaret immediately rectified the miscommunication over the plain rice and then found that the same issue was plaguing the patients over at the burn center. She went to visit them and explained that they were not being shown any form of disrespect but that it was simply a misunderstanding of cultures. She promised to speak with the hospital kitchen staff and then showed the cooks how to prepare Nigerian-style rice-and-meat stew using cayenne pepper, tomato sauce, and a plentiful helping of beef or fish. The next meal served at both hospitals was morale raising for the patients.

This informative interaction with the dietitians prompted the cooks to become more creative with other recipes, and mealtime became a highlight at both hospitals. I noted the Nigerians with burns on their faces showed their appreciation by managing small twisted smiles when food trays were placed before them.

A small smile given at a time when millions of bacteria were still ravaging their bodies was a hopeful sign. If the majority of burn patients were still able to smile by the end of the week—*if only* . . . I paused. Was I asking for a miracle?

CHAPTER 17

Ann Arbor: One Week Later

It was the first full week of patient treatment at the burn center, and we were nearing the end of the emergent period and entering what is called the *acute period*, the second phase of burn treatment. During this period, the burn team has two major tasks: first is caring for the wound by removing the dead tissue in areas of full-thickness skin loss, followed by autografting, replacing the skin with tissue from the skin bank; second is managing infections and metabolic complications. The patient remains in this acutely ill category until all skin grafting has been completed. For severe burns like those the Nigerians had sustained, the hazardous acute period would require weeks to months of treatment.

Early in the acute period, when two of the more seriously burned young Nigerian men, both casual workers, were first taken to the water bath to clean their burn wounds in preparation for skin grafting, their eyes widened in anxiety as the burn staff prepared to lower them into the tubs of water. To them the water bath environment looked more like a morgue than a healing center. In the Nigerian culture, those judged too severely burned to survive were given medicines to erase the pain while they were eased into a more comfortable death. Fearful that the Americans had decided to end their lives by sedating them and drowning them in the bubbling water tubs, the two young men with hideous burns screamed and savagely fought to escape. The words they shouted were unrecognizable to the burn staff. In the ensuing skirmish, they kept screaming the same monosyllable words over and over, forcefully pointing at the exit to the bath facility.

It was apparent to the burn center staff that the two patients hadn't understood that the water baths were not only safe but also an absolutely essential component of the treatment regimen. To terminate the brawl, the two panicking Nigerians were calmed by smiling personnel slowly speaking simple English words to inform them that the water baths were one of the best ways to clean their burned skin in preparation for skin grafting. More importantly, the frequent water bath treatments would shorten the time they would have to remain in a situation they feared, not knowing the real reason for the bath treatments.

This traumatic episode alerted the staff to the fact that there might be a communication impediment they hadn't known existed. While all the Nigerians did speak English, it was not their primary language, and in their condition, many were unable to communicate as well as they might have in perfect health. In addition, there were many different dialects among the patients, so reliance on plain

English was not the best way to communicate. It was essential that the Nigerian patients become better informed participants in their surgical and medical treatments and that this communication barrier featuring five Nigerian dialects—Yoruba, Efik, Ibo, Hausa, and Ghanian—had to be overcome. But how?

Margaret had been fully cognizant of this cultural and language barrier from the beginning and offered to help overcome the meal problems. She also assisted members of the burn staff to recruit help from the surprisingly large number of Nigerian students attending the University of Michigan. In total, forty-three students, and their significant others, willingly joined in the communication and morale-boosting efforts at the burn center. The Nigerian students knew the various dialects spoken by the patients and graciously served as interpreters. I observed that as a group, the Nigerian students were anxious to do what they could to allay the fears of their countrymen.

One Nigerian couple studying at the university became the lead coordinators for the other students, establishing a visitation schedule. Another couple, working closely with the hospital dietitians, arranged for the students who wished to bring Nigerian-style food to the patients at mealtime to do so. In addition to rice, traditional Nigerian cuisine includes vegetables such as yams and peppers, cornmeal, nut oils, and legumes. When the students arrived with their food, morale among the patients was immediately boosted. In addition, these frequent visitations cultivated friendships and allowed the patients to be regularly updated on the latest news from their home country. Those who were still heavily bandaged were also assisted in writing letters back to their family and friends in Nigeria. Most importantly, this comradeship helped the burn patients cope with the emotional shock their hideous burns and scars overwhelmed them with each time they looked in the mirror.

The pinnacle of success was reached two weeks later when Margaret and the students, with the permission of the medical staff, introduced the burn patients to American ice cream, milkshakes, and fast-food hamburgers.

Thus, the communication crisis ended. The staff-and-patient relationships became warm, informative, and comfortable from then on.

It was around this time that a leading Nigerian journalist was visiting the United States and was to be honored at a dinner party given at a premiere hotel in Milwaukee. Because of the role I played in the rescue of the burn victims, I was invited to attend the event. I was enjoying all the festivities until the journalist, during a break, took me aside and admonished me for our intervention in the burn victims' fate—she believed they should be allowed to die a quiet, quick death. She said that all those who survived would be shunned once they returned to their home country, they would be unemployable, they would never marry, and they would live the rest of their lives as though in a nightmare of isolation and rejection. She said that they would be better off as lepers—at least then they would die an early death. Surviving burn victims in her home country, she told me, don't have the luxury of hastened death.

I was absolutely taken aback by this woman's adamant beliefs. I told her that one of the best plastic surgeons in the world would attend to the burn scars and that

Johnson–Nigeria would certainly allow the burn patients to return to work once they had fully recovered. They certainly wouldn't be ostracized, I tried to assure her.

She told me quite loudly to forget it, that it would never happen, that no matter how good the plastic surgery, they would now join the ranks of the pathetic lepers! She said that even if Nigeria–Johnson allowed them to work, they would still be outcasts, that all the other workers would avoid them like the plague. She continued on, asking me if I could imagine the reception they would receive when they tried to go shopping. Storekeepers, she said, would point to the door and shout, calling them lepers and telling them to never come back.

I was devastated by these remarks. The series of multiple skin grafting procedures interspersed with plastic surgeries to minimize the burn scars could be a major hurdle difficult for anyone to leap over. Dr. Feller's plastic surgery skills would have to be impeccably great to allow most of these patients to return to a happy, normal life in Nigeria.

CHAPTER 18

A Visitor from Nigeria:
Ann Arbor—July and August

Chief Jonathan Adio Obafemi Olopade flew to the United States from Nigeria on Monday, July 12, to visit the burn patients, several of whom were members of his tribe. He also wanted to meet with me and those at SC Johnson who were involved in the rescue operation, though I had to decline the invitation due to an out-of-town commitment.

July was a hectic month for me. I was overseeing my medical directorship and product toxicology responsibilities at SC Johnson. Furthermore, I was busy with weekly experiments on the potentially toxic agents in human exposure chambers and scheduled lectures at the Medical College of Wisconsin. The half days and weekend hours I did manage to free up were spent in Ann Arbor at the burn center, observing the treatment and recovery of the ten surviving Nigerian patients.

SC Johnson had a helicopter waiting at Chicago O'Hare International Airport to transport Chief Olopade to Racine, where he was taken to the Council House, the exclusive SC Johnson hotel for premiere visitors. That evening the chief had cocktails and dinner at the Council House with Sam Johnson and nine other top executives, including Ray Farley and Bob Peterson. The next morning, Chief Olopade toured the Johnson complex that included the Biology Center, Wingspread, and the Golden Rondelle Theater, where he viewed the films *Living Planet*, *To Fly*, and *To Be Alive*. These films were for employees and visitors to enjoy and were relevant to the facility as they dealt with personal health, the history of the company, and the philosophy of SC Johnson. The chief had lunch with the executives, many of whom were in the manufacturing services overseas, as well as safety, equal opportunity, and employee relations. After lunch, the chief was given a tour of Waxdale—the name given to the sprawling manufacturing complex—the medical center, and the business area outside SC Johnson headquarters.

That evening the chief was invited to the Council House for a dinner in honor of the ambassador of France to the United Nations, His Excellency M. Luc de La Barre de Nanteuil. After breakfast the next morning, the chief was flown to Ypsilanti, Michigan, a city adjacent to Ann Arbor, and on to the burn center for a leisurely visit with the Nigerian patients.

On Tuesday, July 13, one additional burn patient, number 5, Samuel Oluwasuyi, lost his life due to an overwhelming bacterial bronchopneumonia. He was twenty-one and had 65 percent of his body burned. Only his chest had been spared. During his hospitalization, doctors were constantly challenged with treating all the complications that developed, including respiratory problems, renal failure, and heart failure. Essentially, every system in his body slowly failed. The clinical cause of death was listed as bilateral bronchopneumonia and sepsis. A cousin was listed as his next of kin. Hearing about this man's death, it struck me that every country in the world should have prompt access to a major burn center—each badly burned world citizen deserved a chance at survival no matter where they came from.

The burn care center's endeavor to save and restore the lives of the remaining burn patients over the next months was a spectacular undertaking to witness. At the time of the death of the eighth burn victim, only two of the ten burn patients on the road to full recovery were Alison Ehiemere and Okon Bassey. This left eight patients whose survival was still questionable.

To my relief, by the following week, a third patient joined the ranks of the probable survivors; and during the last three weeks of July, the number of definite survivors crept up to four—then eight—and finally all ten!

Over the months to come, the eight survivors with the largest areas of full-thickness skin loss would undergo multiple surgeries for debridement of the eschar in order to prepare a clean surface of granulation tissue for skin grafts, initially homografts from the donor bank and followed by autografts of the patient's own skin as it became available. The homografts, though temporary, are considered lifesaving and seal the wound, protecting it from bacterial invasion. In approximately one month, the body rejects most homografts; but in the meantime, a small autograft has time to heal and present a healthy skin surface that can be used to provide additional autografts. The tedious skin grafting can take months before all the burn areas in a person with 30 to 90 percent total body full-thickness skin burns are protectively covered with his or her own skin.

As skin grafting nears completion, the patient enters rehabilitation. For the severely traumatized patient, rehabilitation includes correction of functional and cosmetic deformities, management of emotional problems, and the continued detection and treatment of any organ system complications. Successful rehabilitation results when all problems are addressed simultaneously and resolved according to a plan individualized for each patient. First, correction of functional deformity is usually accomplished by helping the patient to return to normal activity; as soon as conditions permit, cosmetic reconstruction, essential for the patient's emotional rehabilitation, should be started.

The emotional and social problems that trouble the burn patient probably constitute the most difficult aspect of the rehabilitation process. This total care program requires the careful management by members of the burn team: the surgeon, nurse, social worker, psychiatrist, and therapist working together to provide the critical psychosocial support. In the case of these particular patients, the psychological support given by Allison, his wife Margaret, and the Nigerian students in Michigan to overcome the cultural and communication barriers was outstanding.

The case of Dele Jacob, the twenty-eight-year-old accounts clerk, is representative of what the other severely burned patients experienced. When Irv and I first saw Dele Jacob at the Ajanaku Hospital on June 24, he was dehydrated, had a high fever, and had not received the appropriate wound cleaning, adequate IV fluids, and antibiotics.

When he first arrived at the burn center, he was alert and cooperative and spoke English quite well. His main complaint was the severe pain in areas where he was burned—mouth, ears, scalp, chest, abdomen, upper extremities, thighs, and upper legs. He did admit that he had had an attack of malaria about three months prior to the burn injuries, but there was no history of prior surgeries or medical problems.

Dele was resuscitated with fluids, given antibiotics, and began the process of wound cleansing and debridement. He did well until June 29, when he suddenly spiked a temperature of 107.5°F and lost consciousness. The medical staff reasoned that most likely he was experiencing an overwhelming infection or possibly another attack of malaria. New antibiotics were immediately administered, and he was immersed in a cold water bath. Shortly after immersion, he regained consciousness and screamed that he wanted to drown and die. Struggling to keep his head submerged in the water, he fought the attendants who were keeping his head above the water level with his fists and feet. Several minutes later, when his temperature dropped a few degrees, he became calmer; and once again he could smile while he shivered and thanked the staff for the water treatment. Malaria was ruled out, and he was given the antibiotics best suited to destroy the bacteria circulating in his blood. Following this stressful episode, the routine daily baths and debridement program resumed.

During July and early August, all of Dele's full-thickness burn wounds were successfully covered with autografts, and the partial-thickness burns were epithelialized—that is, his own body created new tissue to cover the wounds. On July 15, surgery was performed with split-thickness skin grafting and a tarsorrhaphy, a surgical procedure where the eyelids are partially sewn together to narrow the opening over the eye. On July 22, he had an operation for a lower-eyelid release and patch grafting in this area. On July 28, small autografts were applied to his hands where he had exposed tendons. These grafts healed adequately by the time of his discharge. It was noted by the staff that he still had a great deal of work to do on increasing the range of motion in his hands. On August 2, the day before his discharge from the burn center to the Chelsea Community Hospital, he complained that his vision was becoming cloudy, and it was evident that he was unable to fully close his eyelids. Thus, a tarsorrhaphy procedure was performed a second time to aid in total eye closure.

It was during this long period of recovery that I had the chance to chat with Dele and learn a bit about his earlier life. He was born in 1954 in Accra, the capitol of Ghana, where his father was a shipping manager, and he grew up with five brothers and three sisters and attended Accraroyar School for three years, studying accounting. In 1977, he met his wife-to-be, Vicentia Quartey, in Accra, and at the time of the Johnson–Nigeria fire incident, they were planning to marry. Dele told me that he only wanted to survive in order to be with Vicentia. Initially, her family objected to the marriage due to Dele's predicament, but Vicentia insisted that she could handle the situation and the two were still planning to be married upon his return to Nigeria.

A Visitor from Nigeria: Ann Arbor—July and August

During the months of July and August, the burn team worked tirelessly to care for the Nigerians, applying skin grafts to all the areas where the burns were full thickness, while warding off the potentially lethal bacterial attacks still threatening their well-being. Thankfully, this was successful, and by the end of August, all the Nigerians were released and returned to Nigeria for a six-month period, to allow their skin grafts to heal and to afford them time with their family and loved ones. The burn team knew full well that while this healing process took place, gruesome scarring would become more and more prevalent—disfiguring scarring that would place these individuals into the ranks of the despicable social outcasts. To avoid this fate, each Nigerian had been told that he could return to the burn center after six months and have the ugly newly formed scars removed, which should allow each person to reenter Nigerian society without the "leper" label.

During this waiting period, I dedicated myself to learning more about skin grafting from *Reconstruction and Rehabilitation of Burned Patients*. While acquiring this knowledge, I decided to focus on Allison's burns as a start. His most serious burns were of full thickness on the entire dorsum of both of his hands and ears. The Feller and Grabb compendium unequivocally stated that of all the areas of the body with full-thickness skin burns, the hand is considered a key area for prompt restoration. Early return of function in the hand not only dramatically enhances the patient's hope for successful rehabilitation but, more importantly, also gives a psychological boost to his or her morale by allowing him or her to become an active participant in his or her own care.

Allison was operated on by Dr. Feller twelve days after his admission to the burn center. First, skin was taken from the back of his thigh and most of it was grafted to his hands, both of which were badly burned. Both ears also required grafting. Once this type of surgery is completed, the hand must be properly elevated and splinted while it heals. If, after surgery, the hand is not splinted, it will become grossly deformed as healing proceeds. In Allison's case, both hands would have resembled claws with thumb and fingers frozen in a state of useless immobility. After surgery and healing, exercises begin until all range of motion is regained.

Okon Bassey was the first and only patient to escape any form of surgery. The burns to his upper extremities were all partial thickness, so he was treated with a routine burn protocol of baths twice a day and frequent dressing of the wounds. His skin infections were treated with the appropriate antibiotics for the repeated spikes of temperature caused by a staph infection. Upon his return to Nigeria, Okon left the Johnson company and started work as a security guard for the Santana Security Company.

Victor Akalona—the twenty-five-year-old casual worker with 47 percent burns, some partial and some deep, over his face, torso, arms and legs—underwent one operation for debridement and split-thickness skin grafting from his right thigh. His left and right ears and his neck also required skin grafts. Complications, such as elevated white blood cell count and anemia, were also successfully treated. Victor was discharged on July 21 and was to have follow-up treatment by a plastic surgeon upon his return to Nigeria. He continued working for Johnson–Nigeria for six months then quit to start his own trading business.

Oli One, the operations manager, underwent one operation for debridement and split-thickness skin grafting of his left eyelid, left forehead, and left ear with skin taken from his thigh. He continued working for Nigeria–Johnson for six months, then quit, and went into the private manufacturing business. He also introduced his own brand of insecticide to the market and is now in the business of supplying chemical raw materials.

CHAPTER 19

The Final Hurdle: Ann Arbor—Nine Months Later

Dele Jacobs said that when he went back to Nigeria for the break between surgeries, people at the Johnson–Nigeria office were shocked. He said when he was out in public, people stared, but not everybody. They wanted to know what happened to him. He told me that they looked at him as if they had never seen a person in that state before. Dele said it was emotionally upsetting, and he had been looking forward to his return to the burn center in March 1983 for the removal of the big scars on his face and body.

When Dele and the other most seriously burned patients returned to the burn center in March 1983 for their follow-up plastic surgeries, they were delighted to learn that during those three months in Michigan, they would be housed at the top floor of a new hotel, just blocks from the center. In addition, Dr. Feller arranged for a special dining room that served only Nigerian-style food, plus a large room in which the Nigerians could meet with friends or watch TV. For morning rounds Dr. Feller had his staff walk with him to the hotel to care for the Nigerians and to oversee their recovery from multiple plastic surgeries. SC Johnson would be charged only $10 per night for each Nigerian instead of the $100 to $200 per night at the Chelsea Community Hospital.

During Dele's four-and-a-half-month stay in Ann Arbor in 1983, he underwent forty-two surgical procedures over the course of six operations. His first surgery, which kept him under anesthesia for nearly three hours, included release of the contractures on his hands and in the webbing of his fingers. Contractures form as burned skin heels and causes the skin, and sometimes tendons, to contract, making it difficult to separate the fingers. Following surgeries focused on releasing the scar contractures on his eyelids and ears, removing the scarring from his hands, repairing the scarring on his cheeks and hands, and finishing touches to all the burned areas on his face and hands.

While these surgeries were in progress, Dele received occupational and physical therapy. He was also involved in a rehabilitation program for both individual and group therapies to assist him in learning how to live with the physical and emotional changes that come with the burn so that he could return to his society and work. He was seen in Dr. Feller's office as an outpatient twenty-three times for follow-up care, which included dressing changes, clip removals, and emotional support. He had medications and equipment to take back to Nigeria with him, including a neck collar and topical ointments. During the burn accident, Dele had lost two front teeth, so he was seen by an associate professor of dentistry, who provided the necessary correction for the problem.

In August 1983, Dele was discharged from the burn center, and in October he returned to work at Johnson–Nigeria for a two-week trial period before returning to work full-time. All went well, and his fellow employees were amazed that his skin looked so normal without the previously hideous scars. The trial period went well, and Dele continued full-time at the plant. After a few weeks, he hurried to Ghana to marry his sweetheart, Vicentia Quartey, now twenty-six years old, who was working at a pharmaceutical company there.

Dele Jacob was the only one of the ten surviving burn victims who continued to work at Johnson–Nigeria, where he rose to become the assistant manager before recently retiring. He and Vicentia have four children: two sons, nineteen and twenty-three, and two daughters, seventeen and fourteen. The family attends the Christ for All Missions Church.

Five others of the seriously burned Nigerians also returned to the burn center in March 1983 for several months of skin graft surgeries. Most of them underwent many surgical procedures—some as many as thirty-one—to replace skin, correct the scarring, and repair other conditions resulting from the burns, as well as to undergo occupational and physical therapy.

As for the other burn victims, Sule Oduwaye, the forty-year-old operator, returned home to his wife and children. He left Johnson–Nigeria to start his own trading business. Micheal Enu, nineteen years old, quit Johnson–Nigeria and moved to Ghana, where he is now married and has three children. He owns a business for trading on motor spare parts and building materials. Emmanuel Adeeko, forty seven years old, returned to Johnson–Nigeria for six months and then left to start a trading business, which has done very well. He is married and has children. Hycenth Munonyi, thirty, quit upon his return to Nigeria, and he also went into a successful trading business. He is married and has children. Friday Ononuwa, thirty two years old, returned home to Nigeria and became self-employed.

Allison Ehiemere, shortly after returning to Nigeria in 1982, resumed his old position as the general manager for Johnson–Nigeria. He was soon transferred to England, where he served for three years as Johnson's area director of Industrial Products Division for Nigeria, Ghana, Kenya, Egypt, and Morocco. In 1983, when Barney Miller retired and Vic Thomas took over as regional director for Africa and the Near East, Allison's position was eventually eliminated due to a business downturn in the region. Vic recommended Allison for a position with the company in Racine, but Allison, now forty-four, opted for early retirement so that he could return to Nigeria and contribute to its development. He set up a small business and sold agricultural chemicals from 1987 to 1991, but he and Margaret soon became aware of "how much things were falling apart in the country," with the closing of schools and the universities his children were attending. The family had little choice but to leave and resettle in Detroit. Margaret had no difficulty resuming her job as a science teacher with tenure in the Detroit Public Schools. Allison took sales jobs with various companies until his retirement fourteen years later: "I was grossly underutilized or underemployed in all positions I held, but I had to persevere."

During these years in Detroit, Allison and Margaret continued helping to support the extended Ehiemere family in Nigeria, aiding those who wanted to establish themselves in a way that enabled them to become independent. Allison said, "We envision that some of our younger relatives who have become professionals and gainfully employed—doctors, engineers, lawyers, accountants, teachers, traders, pharmacists—will, in turn, be able to help other still younger family members coming behind them."

Margaret and Allison were honored with chieftaincy titles by their community, Nsulu Ancient Kingdom, in 2005. In appreciation, the two promised to do more for Nsulu in the future. To stay true to this promise, in 2007, Allison established the charitable nonprofit Care Africa Inc. to promote improvement in medical and educational services in Africa, particularly Nigeria, by sourcing and distributing medical and educational supplies and equipment.

Metropolitan Detroit awarded Margaret their Distinguished Service Award for Outstanding Selfless Devotion to science education. She served on the school board for nine years and as president in 2000. She ran workshops in astronomy as a teacher resource agent of the American Astronomical Association, as well as workshops for the Science Education for Public Understanding Project (SEPUP), a project she plans to introduce in Nigeria. She was also inducted into the National Association of Negro Business and Professional Women in spring 2010.

In her church parish, Margaret is secretary of the committee that organizes monthly mass in the Igbo language—Allison's native language—in hopes that such a mass gives their grandchildren an opportunity to experience the culture of their grandfather in a supportive social group.

The story of these ten badly burned but ultimately triumphant Nigerians who survived the terrifying explosion and were able to return to a normal existence is an important tale for the annals of history. For an American company to adhere to the codes of human decency as SC Johnson did was a first in the history of U.S. businesses in Africa. Being a part of this heroic effort has given me hope in the goodness of people, such as Sam Johnson, Jim Keane, Bob Petersen, Barney and Diana Miller, Vic Thomas, and Allison and Margaret Ehiemere, who were guided by the principles of SC Johnson's business philosophy and their own moral and religious ideals. This story, if it can stand as an example of anything, is an example that mankind is capable (and, hopefully, ready to embrace) the basic principle of human decency: *Treat your neighbor as you would have him or her treat you, always remembering that your neighbor is any human being who needs your help.*

AFTERWORD

My 1982 medical adventure in Nigeria introduced me to a fantastic group of individuals who used their talents to save the lives of the severely burned Nigerians. Now I wish to tell you what I have learned about their lives since then. The actions of the people in this story tell us that they are guided by the same basic principles of life: treat your neighbor as you would have him or her treat you, always remembering that your neighbor is any human being who needs your help.

James F. Keane, who launched this rescue mission, left the company in March 1986 due to personal and family business commitments requiring him to relocate to the New York area. He had been with SC Johnson since 1974. He passed away seven or eight years ago.

L. Robert "Bob" Peterson, who responded to Keane's request for a physician and medical supplies and who approached me for the task, retired in 1986 (after having worked at SC Johnson since 1947) and moved to Arizona. A fine golfer, he still plays at age eighty-six and recently spent some of the summer months playing golf in Racine, Wisconsin.

Raymond Farley retired from SC Johnson in 1990. Now eighty-five, he remains an active member of the Johnson Mutual Benefit Association and serves as a trustee of Northwestern University.

Victor Awadagin Thomas retired from SC Johnson in January 1999 at age fifty-seven. He established a trust in Nigeria aimed at assisting students who have entered medical school but who are unable to finish their studies due to lack of funds. Entirely funded by the Thomas family, the Horatio Oritsejolomi Thomas Trust is named after Vic's late father, who felt passionately about medical education. Vic has been closely involved with a charitable organization in England called the Birmingham Settlement, which was established over one hundred years ago to offer opportunities for people held back by either disadvantage or discrimination.

Vic has also written a guidebook for starting business in African countries and is working on a novel about the increasing disparity that exists between the world's haves and have-nots. On a lighter note, Vic participated with a neighbor in a classic car rally, driving from London to Beijing through twelve countries, in a 1958 Morris Minor that came in third in its class.

Vic and his wife, Jean, continue to have adventures in all parts of the world.

Barney Miller retired from SC Johnson in 1983 so he could devote more of his time to the things in life that he embraced and loved the most: his family, music, theater, swimming, and helping those who desperately needed his financial aid.

Until age seventy-three, Barney regularly performed children's puppet shows while living in Argentina to raise money for children's charities. He continued the shows in England for bilingual audiences. Currently, Barney puts on shows, plays his guitar, and sings. In 2003, he served as chairman of the Young Artists Trust, which offers management assistance to classical musicians after they have graduated from a music college, and was also the vice chairman of the United Kingdom Academy of Tango.

Barney organized conferences with the British and Argentineans to build bridges between the British and the Falkland Islanders. He became chairman of the Anglo-Argentine Society in London. On May 20, 1993, Barney received a letter from the Foreign and Commonwealth Office in London, informing him that the Queen had appointed him the Most Excellent Order of the British Empire (OBE) for his valuable contribution to Anglo-Argentine relations over the years. Barney elected to receive the OBE from the British ambassador in Argentina. In November 2008, Barney became chairman of the Anglo-Argentine Society in London for the second time. The society now has seven hundred members.

Barney continues as an active fund-raiser for BABS (British-American Benevolent Society) in Buenos Aires, Argentina, which funds a retirement home on the outskirts of Buenos Aires. Eighty-five residents, some of whom have fallen on hard times and are unable to continue paying the rising rental premiums, are now subsidized by Barney's fund-raising with musical performances.

Additionally, Barney's love for swimming had led to his swimming five days a week. In 2004, at age seventy-six, he and his brother swam from the Isle of Wight to the mainland and from Alcatraz to San Francisco. In 2009, at age seventy-nine, Barney competed with 120 other swimmers in a two-mile swimming contest.

Barney and wife Diana currently live in Chelsea, England.

Dr. Irving Feller retired in 1990 after helping to make the University of Michigan Trauma Burn Center into a nationally known first-class facility. He planned to spend time on the sixty-acre farm he and his wife Cynthia owned adjacent to a state park on the outskirts of Chelsea, Michigan, which they remodeled from an old barn into a spectacular home with many unique features from structures they had seen in Bali, one of the three thousand smaller Indonesian islands the two of them were visiting each year. But always the entrepreneur, Feller and his wife began selling honey-cured smoked capons for Thanksgiving and Christmas and this became so profitable they eventually sold the land and the farm to a private developer who turned it into an upscale suburban community.

The University of Michigan Medical Center Trauma Burn Center, following its success in saving the lives of the severely burned Nigerian employees, was gifted money by Sam Johnson to enlarge the center. On the wall at the entrance to a major research section was a plaque that reads, "The Johnson's Wax Fund Burn Research Laboratories." In 2009, the plaque was changed to read, "SC Johnson Burn Research Laboratories." Adding to the Johnson contribution, another gift from the Kellogg Foundation—plus money from the University of Michigan—dramatically expanded the burn center, which now occupies the whole area on the floor above the emergency room.

In September 1986, a new burn center was opened at the University of Michigan. It was designed by the staff from the "old" burn center based on their twenty-eight years of experience in the care of burned patients under the direction of Dr. Irving Feller. After Dr. Feller retired, Dr. Jai Prasad was named burn director. The steady advancement in burn care research and therapy continues under his leadership.

By 1991, the burn center dramatically expanded its operations by including specialized care for severely injured trauma patients, and the center was renamed the University of Michigan Trauma Burn Center. In 1994, the TBC began its Injury Prevention and Outreach programs.

The Trauma Burn Center's Skin Bank was accredited by the American Association of Tissue Banks in 1995. For six years this was among the largest banks in the world, and it trained representatives from other skin and tissue banks from throughout Michigan and the United States as well as Egypt, Spain, China, and Japan. From 1995 through 2000, the TBC researchers developed new techniques for culturing and growing human skin grafts.

In 2001, *In an Instant*, a burn-prevention video, was distributed throughout the world and became a multiple-award winner. In 2002, it won the CINE Golden Eagle National Award for Best Nontheatrical Film and was a finalist in the New York Film Festival.

Today, the TBC is an 8,799-square-foot unit with sixteen beds (ten intensive care and six acute care) to which an average of 1,400 injured patients are admitted each year. The TBC has its own operating room, a wound debridement suite, a skin bank and laboratory, an outpatient clinic, a family activity room, the Med Inn (hotel connected to University Hospital), access to Ronald McDonald House, and additional adult and pediatric intensive care units within the center. Transport services feature three survival flights, twin-engine Bell 430 helicopters, a fixed-wing Cessna citation jet, a mobile intensive care unit, and ground transportation.

The TBC is staffed by three core burn surgeons, including the burn director Dr. Stewart Wang, MD, PhD, who is also the director of the Program for Injury Research and Education. The TBC is verified as both a burn center and a level 1 trauma center by the American Burn Association and the American College of Surgeons. To be considered verified, a center must demonstrate leadership in research, education, outreach, prevention, system planning, and the ability to care for the most severely injured patients. The University of Michigan TBC is one of only fifty-five verified burn centers in the United States. Verification as a burn center and level 1 trauma center is a prestigious accomplishment that the TBC is proud to have attained.

ACKNOWLEDGMENTS

For this biography I thank my wife, Mary, for her amazing support in allowing me to devote a major portion of our life together to serve as a professor of internal medicine and medical toxicology at the Medical College of Wisconsin, to devote my free time to medical research, and the occasional medical adventure to a distant land. I am one lucky doctor to have married such a beautiful, vivacious lady.

Marian Betancourt, my agent, deserves my thanks for her patience in helping me compose this biography for the general public, as well as for the doctors and nurses I had focused on. She knew exactly what to say while avoiding confusing medical terminology.

Dr. Irving Feller, Barney Miller, Robert Peterson, Victor Thomas, and Raymond Farley are the six who not only accomplished this Nigerian rescue mission but also spent the time to allow me to learn about their lives before and since this once-in-a-lifetime medical adventure.

BIBLIOGRAPHY AND NOTES

Bodeau, P. S. *Johnson Wax (Nigeria) Ltd. Accident, June 21, 1982. Time Sequence of Events.* Official SC Johnson Company Report, July 29, 1982.

Feller, Irving. "Survival of a Severely Burned Child." *The Surgical Clinics of North America* 39 (1959): 407–420.

Feller, Irving, and C. Archambeault. *Nursing the Burned Patient.* Ann Arbor, Michigan: The Institute for Burn Medicine, Press of Braun-Brumfield, 1973.

Feller, Irving, and W. C. Grabb. *Reconstruction and Rehabilitation of the Burned Patient.* Dexter, Michigan: The National Institute for Burn Medicine, Press of Thomson-Shore, Inc., 1979.

Feller, Irving, and R. C. Hendrix. "Clinical Pathologic Study of Sixty Fatally Burned Patients." *Surgery, Gynecology & Obstetrics* 119 (June 1964): 1–5.

Feller, Irving, C. A. Jones, and K. Richards. *Emergent Care of the Burn Victim*. Ann Arbor, Michigan: The National Institute for Burn Medicine, 1977.

The Editor: "An Interview with Samuel C. Johnson." *Cornell Executive Graduate School of Management, Cornell University* (Summer/Fall 1983): 4–10.

Johnson, H. F. "This We Believe." *SC Johnson Code of Ethics*, 1927.

Lipman, Jonathan. *Frank Lloyd Wright and the Johnson Wax Buildings*. New York: Rizzoli International Publications, Inc., 1986.

ABOUT THE AUTHOR

Storytelling, American literature, and medical mysteries are the loves of Dr. Richard Stewart, a certified specialist in both internal medicine and medical toxicology, who has devoted most of his medical career to teaching and research at the Medical College of Wisconsin since 1966.

A longtime admirer of Sir Frederick Treves—the famous British physician who turned to writing for the general public in the twilight of his career—Dr. Stewart began a similar journey when he served as director and cohost on station WFMR, Milwaukee's classical music station, for a program that explored the influence of medicine and disease on the lives of famous persons. This avocation prompted his enrollment as a part-time graduate student in English at the University of Wisconsin–Milwaukee to equip himself for writing for the general public. The *Leper Priest of Molokai, the Father Damien Story*, published by the University of Hawaii Press in 2000, is the first of his medical biographies.

Dr. Stewart is a fellow of the American College of Physicians, a fellow of the American College of Clinical Toxicology, and one of the select group of scientists to be named a Fellow of the American Academy of Toxicological Sciences. He has written more than 250 scientific papers, three of which have won awards, and he has served as editor and contributor to *Practice of Medicine*, vol. 9, and *Clinical Medicine*, vol. 12 (Harper & Row). He holds several medical patents, including the hollow fiber artificial kidney; and he led the medical team that pioneered the use of this lifesaving device that was used in 2009 by more than one million persons worldwide.

Currently, he is devoting the majority of his time to polishing the multiple manuscripts he has drafted over the past twenty years—historical novels that reflect the practice of medicine, medical biographies, medical thrillers, and, if time permits, children's stories loved by his grandchildren.